W9-ABT-988

Healing Chakra

Light to Awaken My Soul

Healing Society

Healing Chakra (Workshop Package)

Light to Awaken My Soul

Copyright©2005 by Ilchi Lee
All rights reserved.
No part of this book may be reproduced
or transmitted in any form whatsoever,
without permission in writing from the publisher.

Design: Soo Jeong In, Eun Kyoung Lee, Dongkuramy
Illustrations: Al Choi, Kyoung Hwa Park

Healing Society, Inc.
7664 W. Lake Mead Blvd. #109
Las Vegas, NV 89128

Web site: www.hspub.com

If you are unable to order this book from your local bookseller,
you may order directly from the publisher.
Call 1-928-204-1106

Library of Congress Control Number: 2005922873
ISBN 1-932843-10-8

Printed in South Korea

Healing Chakra

Light to Awaken My Soul

ILCHI LEE

Healing Society

We have come to the Earth
To experience the flowering of our soul,
Rising from our upper Dahn-jon,
Blossoming from the Seventh Chakra.
Who has seen this flower?

Beautiful flower of our soul...
Humans have endured endless suffering,
Long nights of despair,
To nurture this flower of Heavenly Transformation.

Flower of Heavenly Transformation...
Only we humans can help the petals unfold.
When it blossoms within each and every heart
We shall herald a new Age of Peace.

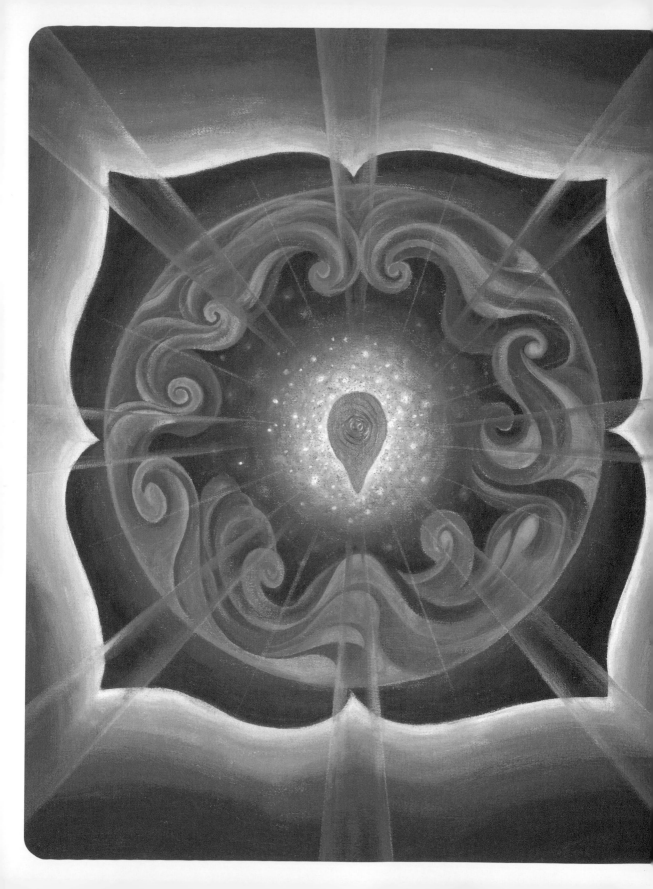

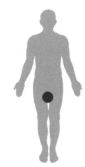

Jade Gate

1ST Chakra

Planted deeply in fertile soil

The flower of life blossoms forth

Providing strength

On which to feed and prosper...

Gate through which we enter the world

Announcing our arrival on Earth

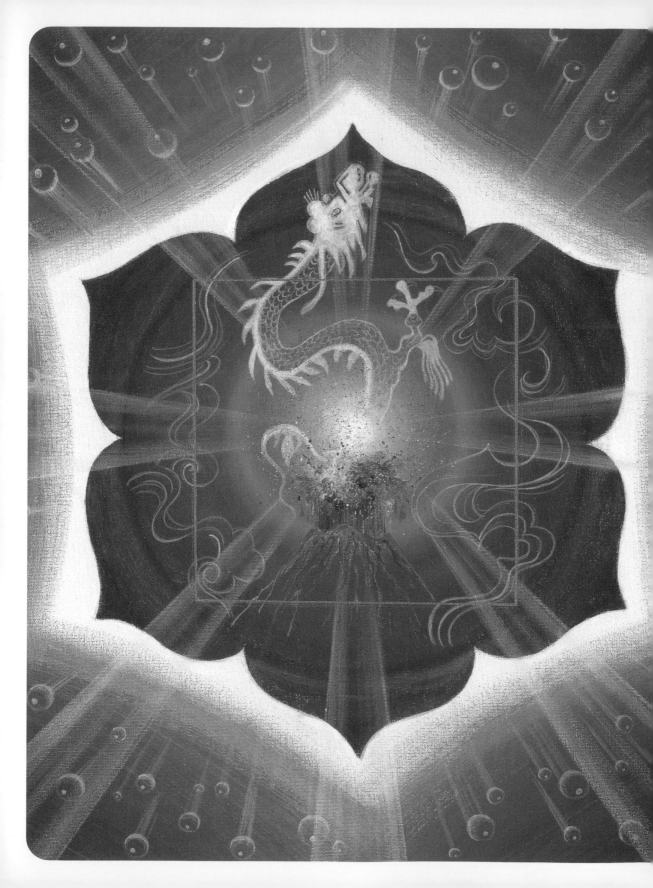

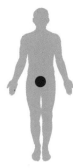

Womb, Earth Palace

2ND Chakra

Earth Palace, nurturing the seed of the physical body

With the rich energy of the Dahn-jon ablaze

Water goes up, and fire comes down

In accordance with the harmonious order of life

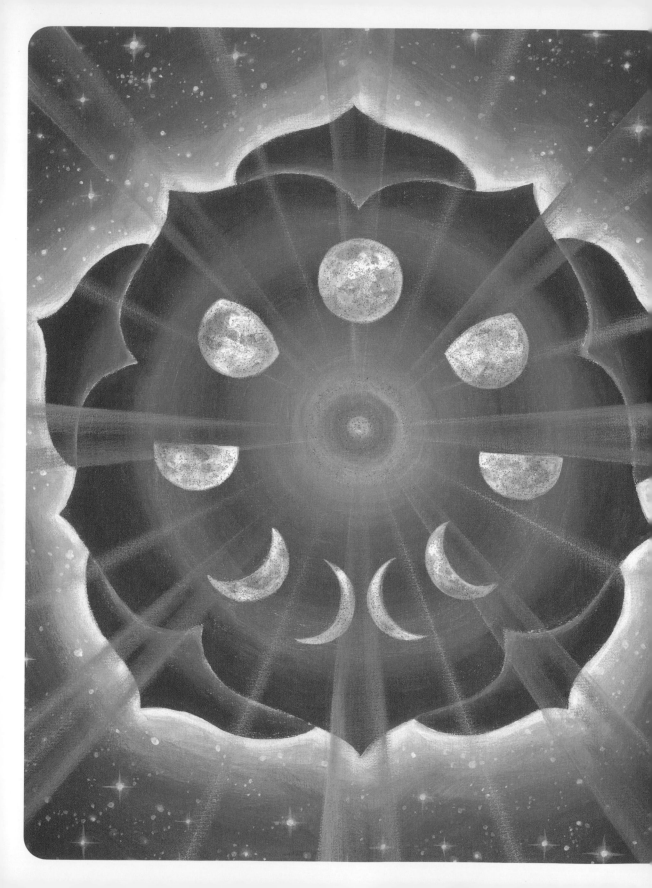

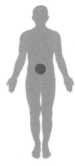

Sun Locus

3RD Chakra

In pink and yellow glory,

A lotus flower in the middle...

Loving, eating, drinking, working, living...

Master of the desire for life

Shining brightly within those who seek

A beautiful life

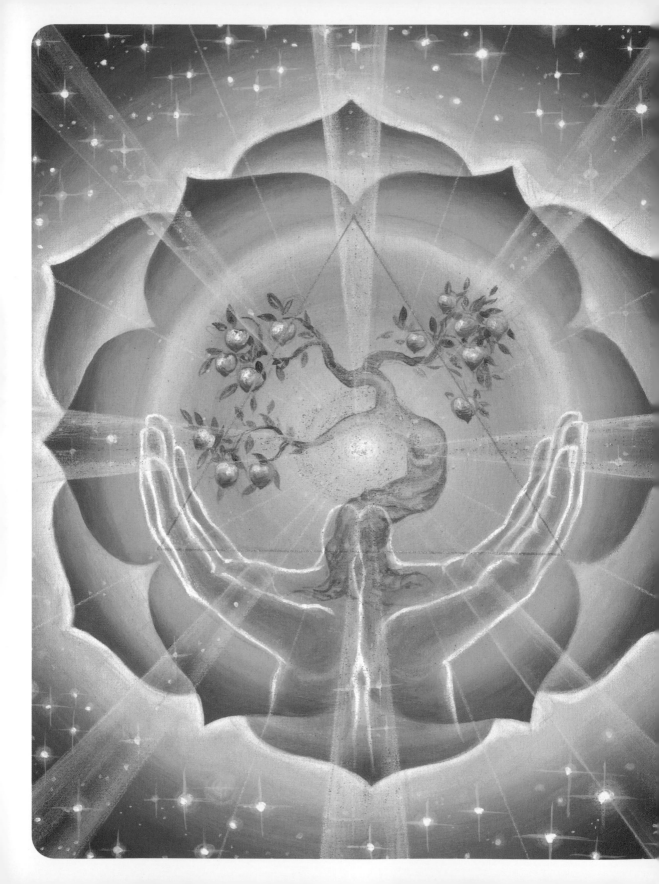

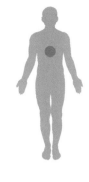

Mind Palace

4ᵀᴴ Chakra

Mind Palace, seat of the soul

Golden lotus, shimmering

Love and compassion residing within

Giving rise to honesty, diligence, responsibility

Coming together with dignity

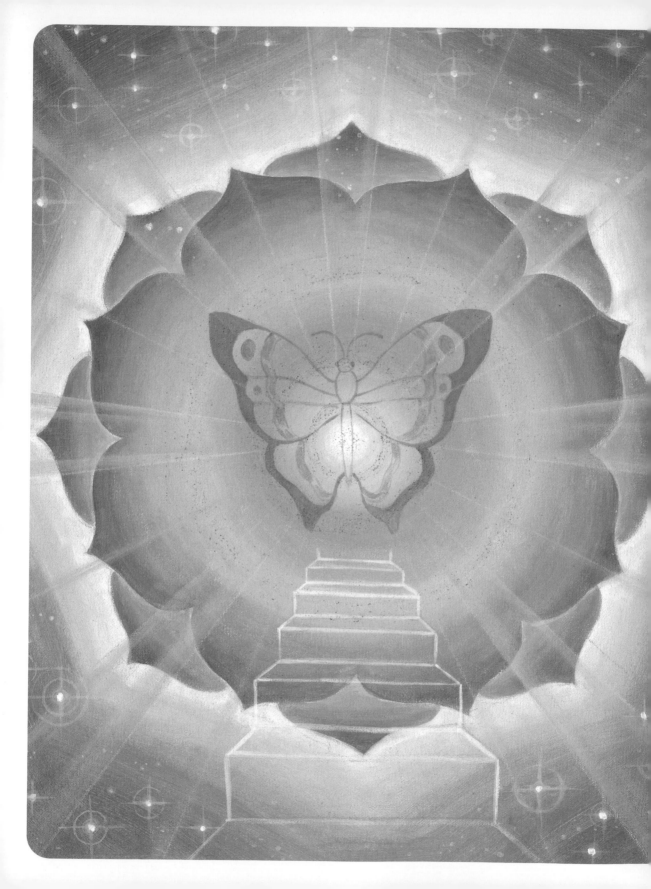

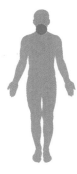

Soul's Gate

5ᵀᴴ Chakra

Gate through which the soul travels

When the blue lotus blooms from the neck

Its azure light connects the Jade Gate

With Heaven's Gate

Allowing advancement of the soul

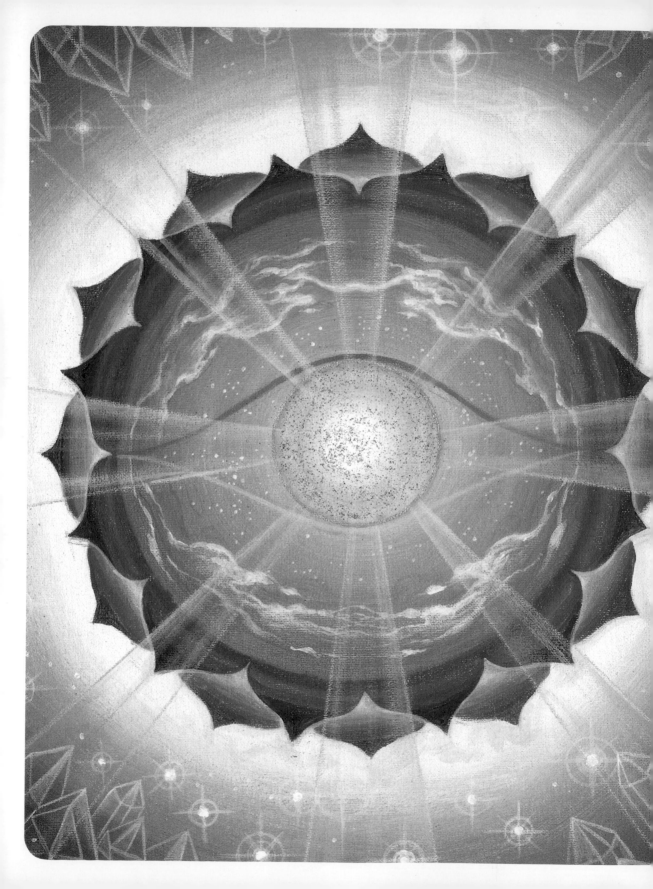

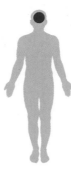

Heaven's Palace

6ᵀᴴ Chakra

Heaven's Palace, source of the rhythm of life, Yullyo...

When the indigo lotus appears upon the In-dang

It awakens the divinity within... our second birth

To life whole and everlasting

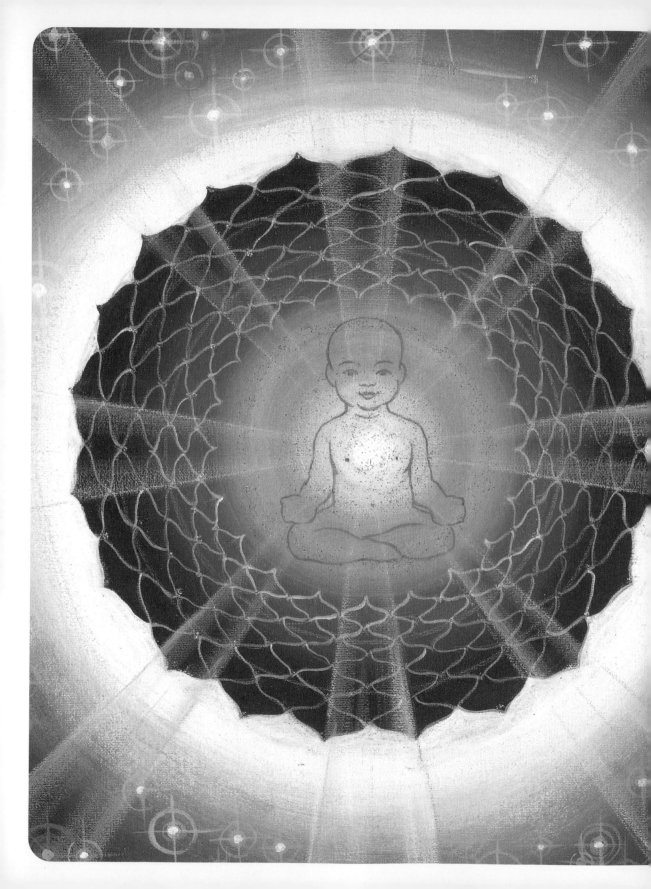

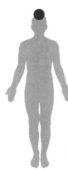

Heaven's Gate

7TH Chakra

Place of our third birth, Heavenly Transformation

Violet lotus rises from the Baek-hwe

Liberating our soul to great freedom

Completing our energy body

Communing with Cosmic Energy

	Location	Spiritual Growth Stage	Characteristics
7TH Chakra Great Heaven's Gate	Baek-hwe (Crown of the head)	Third Birth, Heavenly transformation, birth of the soul, completion of the soul, human divinity, unity, oneness	Transcends time and space, unity of divinity and true self, wisdom and insight
6TH Chakra Heaven's Palace	In-dang (Upper Dahn-Jon, Third Eye)	Second Birth, recognition of divinity within, soul	Enlightenment of the soul, intuition and insight, peace of mind and heart
5TH Chakra Soul's Gate	Throat (Thyroid glands)	Gate separating external and internal strength	Trust, sincerity, and faith; peace with gentleness; balance and harmony
4TH Chakra Mind Palace	Dahn-joong (Sternum)	Conscience, human character	Compassion, forgiveness, understanding, passion, honesty, diligence, responsibility
3RD Chakra Sun Locus	Joong-wahn (Above navel)	Completion of physical health	Self-control, will, discipline, desire for power and authority, warmth, happiness, need for recognition
2ND Chakra Earth Palace	Lower Dahn-jon	Place of physical growth and nurturing	Health, desire, joy, passion, emotions, sexual needs
1ST Chakra Jade Gate	Hwe-um (Perineum)	First Birth, physical birth.	Success, patience, acknowledgment, courage

Color	Anatomical Correspondence	Function	Signs of Problems
Lavender Purple	Neo-Cortex	Activation of the Neo-Cortex	Confusion, early senility, lack of inspiration
Navy blue	Brain Stem	Activation of the brain stem	Lack of concentration, tension, headaches, problems with eyesight, nightmares, overactive cynicism
Blue-green	Thyroid glands, throat	Voice, speaking skills	Lack of conversation or speech skills, ignorance, depression, non-discernment, incorrect use of knowledge, thyroid disease
Gold	Sternum, heart	Circulation, muscle strength; connects life force with True Self	Repression of love, emotional instability, lack of balance, problems with heart/circulation
Orange	Stomach	Metabolism, digestion, emotional stability	Lack of desire for life, fear, hatred, problems with liver and stomach
Soft Red	Uterus, sexual organs, prostate glands	Birth, sexual energy, physical strength, vigor	Loss of appetite for food and sex, lack of life purpose, jealousy, gynecological problems
Dark Red	Intestine, spine, bones	Excretion, life force, survival instinct, self-protection	Selfishness, anxiousness, criminal intent, rage, problems with the spine, chronic constipation

The Road to True Happiness, Peace, and Health

This book was not written to convey
Special or esoteric knowledge.
Everyone seeks happiness and peace in life.
But how do you attain happiness and peace?
Before you can speak of happiness and peace,
You must have health.
This book is intended as a guide to true health,
Happiness, and peace.

Contrary to general belief,
Health is not limited to the physical body.
Our bodies are composed of physical,
Energy and spiritual bodies.
We will become masters of a truly happy and peaceful life
Only when our physical, energy and
Spiritual bodies come together in healthy harmony.
To help us create and maintain harmony among the three bodies,
We have seven precious gems of energy.
These are the seven Chakras.

Chakras are central points for the interchange
Of energy flow in our bodies.
Problems with the Chakras translate into problems
For the body, mind, and spirit.
A change in the Chakras signifies transformation

Of body and mind.
It is not an overstatement to say that complete health begins
And ends with the Chakras.

Are you happy?
This is akin to asking, "Are your Chakras healthy?"
Are you at peace?
This is also like asking, "Are your Chakras healthy?"

This book has been designed to teach you
How to control and transform energy.
Energy is the root of body and mind.
By understanding and mastering energy,
We can unlock the secret to changing ourselves and the world.
When a Chakra changes, energy changes.
When energy changes, personal transformation is achieved.
Transformed people will transform society.

The Heavenly Code is one of the oldest
And most sacred texts in the history of the world.
It has been handed down to us through Korean tradition,
And states that heaven and earth exist within the human,
Signifying that heaven, earth, and humans are all interconnected.
This means that when humans change,
Heaven and earth also change.

If you observe the world and examine humans,
Applying the principles of energy flow,
Then all problems can be solved.
Illness in the body begins
When energy flow becomes unbalanced and disharmonious.
When the human body and the world are diagnosed
From the viewpoint of energy,
It is possible to pinpoint areas of imbalance and correct them.

Healing Chakra training is a way to restore balance
And harmony to our body's Chakra System.
It is also a way to restore the energy balance
Between humanity and today's world.
When you know the Chakras,
You will know health, happiness, and peace.
You will even know the truth of life and the universe.

Ilchi Lee

Contents

Part II Energy and the Body

Part III Healing Chakra Exercises

Contents

Part IV Everyday Healing Chakra

1. Chakra Brain Respiration 116

2. Exercises to Awaken the Chakras 126

Change Your Energy

Change Your Brain

Change Your Life

Part I

Secret of the Golden Flower

True Spiritual Power is Peace

One with a Heart of Peace

.Is One Who has Experienced

The Golden Flower of the Soul...

1. Seven Hidden Gems of the Body

The Secret Tradition of Chakra Healing

Flowing within our bodies is the energy that drives and maintains our life functions. This energy flows not only within our bodies, but also through the very fabric of the universe. In the Orient, we call this energy "Ki," "Chi," or "Prana." There are seven major points of intersection for the flow of this energy in our bodies. These points are called Chakras, or in the Korean tradition, Dahn-jons.

Chakra, a Sanskrit word, means a wheel or a circle. This is because energy tends to swirl in a circular motion as it gathers in the Chakras. In the ancient Asian mind-body-spirit discipline of Shin Sun Do (Way of the Divine), Chakras are called Dahn-jons. Literally translated, Dahn-jon means "field where energy gathers."

Knowledge of the Chakras has long been important in the Vedas and Yoga of India, as well as other Asian traditions. Due to the importance of this knowledge to spiritual traditions of the East, and to the exclusivity of transmission of this information, the Chakras may have been a bit over mythologized. They have been relegated to the realm of the fantastic and have become inaccessible to the average person.

Even in the Korean Shin-Sun-Do tradition, only a very few, select individuals were lucky enough to find a teacher to guide them. In this tradition, "Small Universe" is the state in which all of the Chakras are activated, all meridians of the body flow freely, and the mind and body become one. "Great Universe" is the state in which cosmic and bodily energy merge into one continuous and conscious flow, allowing discovery of the True Self.

A similar philosophy is expressed in Kundalini Yoga. This tradi-

▼ A picture from "Sung-Myung-Ji-Gwe," a 16ᵀᴴ Century book on the practice of Shin-Sun-Do. The pathways of the "Great Universe" - various Dahn-jons or Chakras - are symbolized by drawings of a pot, crescent moon, and stars, among others.

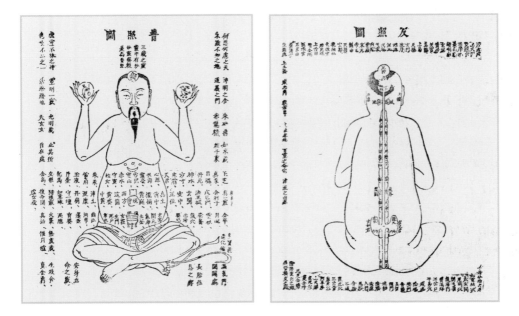

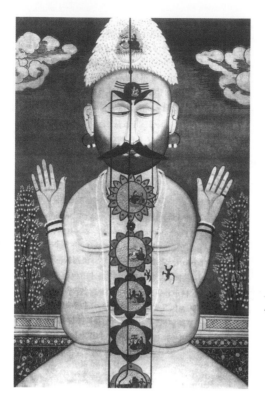

◀ A representation of Chakras from a Yoga tradition. Each tradition has a slightly different interpretation and description of the Chakras.

tion was similarly limited to a very select group of individuals. Kundalini means "life energy coiled in the shape of a snake at the bottom of the spine." It is said that when the coiled life energy awakens, the energy will travel up the spine through the Chakras and effect a spiritual awakening.

Chakras have an intimate relationship with the spiritual growth of a person. To experience and understand the Chakras means that you understand the flow of life, including the meaning of life and death. You might posses the most precious of gems, yet, if you don't know its value, then there is no difference between the gem and an ordinary pebble. One of the primary reasons that people are in constant search for "meaning" in life is that they don't understand the Chakra system within their own bodies. Understanding the True Self, and thereby life's meaning and purpose, lies in an understanding of the Chakras. Experiencing the Chakras will bring about an overall understanding of life.

In the ancient Asian mind-body-spirit discipline of Shin-Sun-Do (Way of the Divine), there is a system for achieving spiritual completion through the Chakras. Healing Chakra training is a modernized version of this ancient system of advancing the spiritual journey, adapted for modern times.

It is with the hope of utilizing this system of Shin-Sun-Do to effectively awaken the potential of the seven Chakras, that I write this book. The name "Healing Chakra" is simply the term I use for this modernized version of traditional Asian Chakra training.

Secrets of Heavenly Transformation of Shin-Sun-Do

In the ancient tradition of Korea, there existed a body-mind-spirit training system called Shin-Il-Hap-Il (Divine-One-Together-One), which sought to elevate human consciousness to its highest plateau, that of divinity. More widely known by the name Shin-Sun-Do, the philosophy and ideas contained therein were originally derived from an ancient sacred text called "Chun-Bu-Kyung," or the Heavenly Code.

The Chun-Bu-Kyung is the highest authority among the sacred texts in Korean spiritual tradition. It is said that the Chun-Bu-Kyung was recorded by an ancient sage who realized his own enlightenment through his training regimen of Shin-Sun-Do, thereby gaining insight into the realities of life and death and the operational flow of the universe. Because the Chun-Bu-Kyung is essentially a numerical representation of the laws of the cosmos, it cannot be interpreted literally. It will only reveal its true nature and meaning to someone who has experienced the realities of life through Ki energy.

When I first realized enlightenment, I did not know that the nature of my enlightenment was already spoken of in the Chun-Bu-Kyung. When I finally had the good fortune to learn of it, I realized that my enlightenment had the same inspiration and source as that of the Chun-Bu-Kyung.

After knowing the Chun-Bu-Kyung, I could sense the energy in each one of its 81 letters when I sank deeply into meditation. The teachings of the Chun-Bu-Kyung came to me not through the intellect, but through actual experience of its energies. When I experienced the oneness of Heaven, Earth, and Human described in the Chun-Bu-Kyung, I felt my body become part of the light of the cosmos, attaining a level of ecstasy and peace that spoke to me of divine blessing.

When we realize our innate divine potential, we become one with the essence of the universe. We become one with creativity, peace and love. Currently in our world, we are trapped in the illusion that we must be in constant competition with one another. We live with the belief that you and I are different and separate. The Chun-Bu-Kyung contains the essence of the trinity, in which good and evil, life and death, heaven and earth are not defined as opposites, but as parts of the same cosmic harmony. When we realize that our essence is identical to the essence that makes up the cosmos, we overcome fear, sadness, and anger.

Oneness, where no barrier exists between you and me, is our

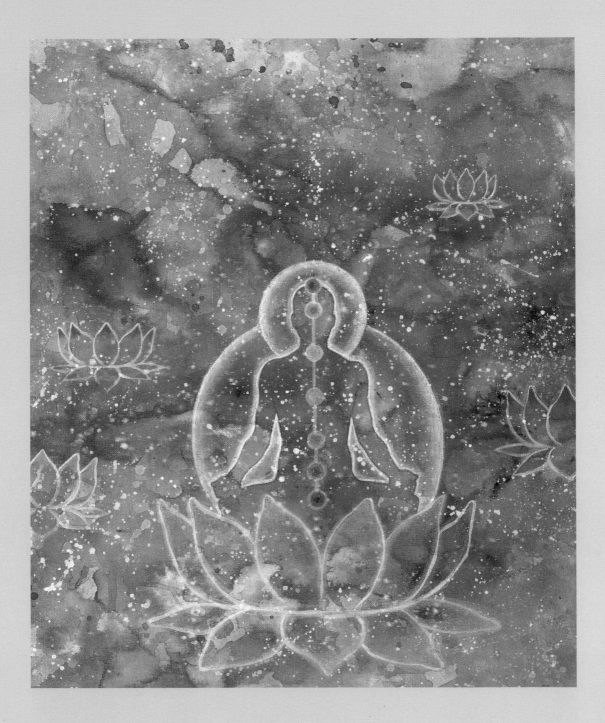

essence and our divinity. As soon as we are born, we begin the struggle to light up this innate divinity. Once we realize our own divine enlightenment, we will achieve Heavenly Transformation. Heavenly Transformation is the process whereby human beings reach the highest level of awareness, and consciously return to the Source at the moment of death. It is this process that is delineated in the letters of the Chun-Bu-Kyung.

The secret to Heavenly Transformation lies in the human brain and Ki energy. The Chun-Bu-Kyung can also be interpreted as a numerical code, outlining the process by which the seven Chakras of the body are activated and made to stimulate the inner potential of the brain in order to achieve spiritual awakening. In order to adapt the ancient discipline of Shin-Sun-Do to the modern era, I choose to focus on the brain and energy.

A spiritual civilization will not come about just because one person attains enlightenment. The whole of humanity must spiritually awaken to the cosmic principles of peaceful co-existence and harmony. *The Chun-Bu-Kyung can act as a guide to lead us across the collective spiritual threshold.*

When the energy system of the body changes, so does consciousness. The state of one's energy is profoundly influenced by the quality and quantity of information in the brain. Therefore, *Brain Respiration*, a training method that focuses on the brain, and *Healing Chakra*, a method that concentrates on the energy system of the body, have a symbiotic relationship. The day our inner spiritual potential flowers through Brain Respiration and Healing Chakra will be the day that heralds the dawn of the Golden Age of Spirituality.

Eternal Life Exists of and by Itself

The key to Healing Chakra is to meet with divinity, the soul. Therefore, the goal of Healing Chakra training is to acknowledge the soul, become consciously aware of its living presence, and act to nurture its growth.

The answers to such questions as: "Why was I born?" "What is my life's purpose?" and "What do I live for?" are already within you. Yet, without knowing our soul, we are prisoners of our own bodies. Since the body is a creature of space and time, it begins to deteriorate and die as soon as it is born. When the body dies off, as it inevitably will, what is left? *The soul.*

Every human being has "divinity" that is of the same essence as the source of the cosmos. Our bodies act as temporary housing for the journey of our souls. We came to the Earth in order to go forward and complete the journey of our soul. Although our physical bodies have their limitations, they also contain the necessary tools to propel our souls toward completion of the journey. These tools are the Chakras and energy. Through the Chakras, we may meet with our soul. Such is the amazing power of our bodies.

Therefore, we are not merely physical beings. Our soul, the essence of our nature, transcends time and space. The soul is eternal life that exists of and by itself. Everyone has this eternal life within. Only when the eyes of your soul open can you recognize the existence of the divinity within. When you realize that you are the essence of eternal life you will be free from fear, loneliness, and grief.

The soul acts through Ki-energy. It is because of the soul that Ki-energy is able to move. You cannot recognize your soul without being sensitized to the flow of Ki. Your body is without value as the vessel of your soul if you don't recognize and utilize Ki-energy to approach your soul. However, since everyone is blessed with Chakras, we can all train, activate, and become consciously aware of our body's energy system. We can then utilize this system to help our soul move forward on its journey.

Healing Chakra is a training to recognize your True Self. Is my body my True Self? Is my soul my True Self? My True Self is my life, divinity, soul, and energy. When you realize that you are eternal, you will realize that life and death are just expressions of the essence of life in different forms. Just as the moon remains essentially the same while its visible shape changes according to where the shadows fall, the essence of life remains the same while its visible shape changes. The sun is beautiful when it rises. It is also beautiful when it sets. Although we cannot see the sun at night, it has not ceased to exist. Our life may seem all too brief when seen from a limited point of view, but actually it is eternal. This is because the underlying reality of life does not change.

For the person who is grounded in the timeless truth of the universe, there is no life and death. He or she can experience eternal joy without being limited by the definitions of good and evil. The essence of Oneness ("Han" in Korean) exists within us. In Korean tradition, this Oneness is called *Yullyo*. Once you recognize the Yullyo within, you will realize the truth about life and the underlying harmony of the cosmos. You will become One with the harmony. Healing Chakra is a training to help you meet the Yullyo within.

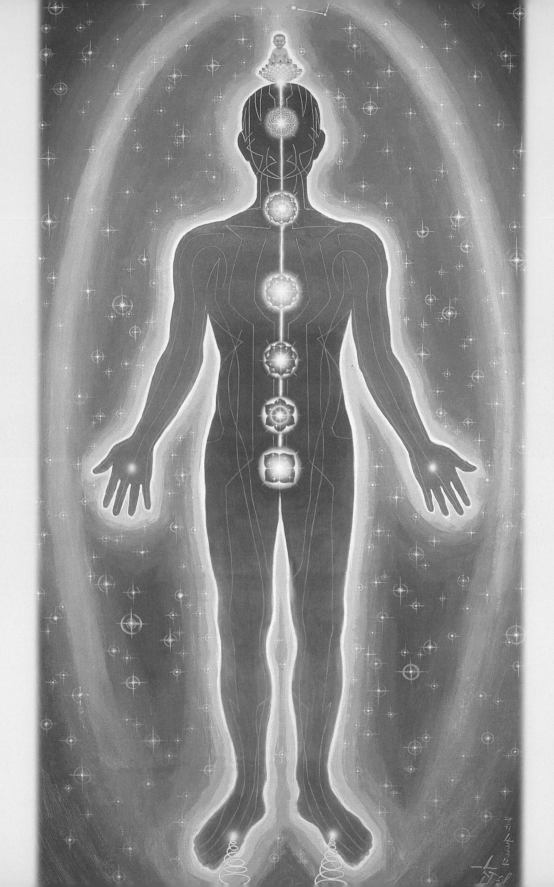

2. Chun-Bu-Kyung (Heavenly Code) and Healing Chakra

Within the letters of the Chun-Bu-Kyung lie the principles and purpose of Healing Chakra. The Heavenly Code can be interpreted as an expression of mathematics, philosophy, and even energy studies. Each letter of the Heavenly Code contains its own distinct letter or numerical meaning when read, and distinct energy or musical characteristics when sounded. It combines number/ratio and sound/energy characteristics of the individual components into a holistic effect, which is an actual representation of the principle of harmonious order. When the effects of the Heavenly Code are applied to the human Chakra system, we can begin to understand the underlying principles of Healing Chakra.

The Heavenly Code describes life as a journey for completion of the soul, a "Way of Heavenly Transformation." This journey of the soul's completion coincides with the activation of the seven Chakras. From the point of view of the "Way of Heavenly Transformation," the seven Chakras consist of three gates and three palaces, giving rise to the third birth in a human life.

天符經

Heavenly Code

一 始 無 始 一 析 三 極 無

盡 本 天 一 一 地 一 二 人

一 三 一 積 十 鉅 無 匱 化

三 天 二 三 地 二 三 人 二

三 大 三 合 六 生 七 八 九

運 三 四 成 環 五 七 一 妙

衍 萬 往 萬 來 用 變 不 動

本 本 心 本 太 陽 昂 明 人

中 天 地 一 一 終 無 終 一

One Begins Unmoved Moving,
That Has No Beginning.
One Divides To Three Crowns,
While Remaining A Limitless Mover.
Heaven Comes First,
Earth Comes Second,
Human Comes Third.
One Gathers To Build Ten,
And Infinite Forms Become The Trinity
(of heaven, earth, human).
Heaven Gains Two To Make Three,
Earth Gains Two To Make Three,
Human Gains Two To Make Three.
Three Trinities Make Six,
And They Create Seven, And Eight, Nine Appears,
And There Comes A Turning.
Three And Four Form A Circle,
Five With Seven Makes One Whole.
Way-Less Is The Way All Comes And All Goes,
Features Are Changing, And Change-Less Is The Maker.
Divine Mind Is Eternal Light,
Looking Toward Celestial Light.
Human Bears Heaven And Earth,
And The Three Make One.

The Principles of Healing Chakra

The Principle of Creation and Evolution

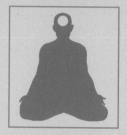

一始無始 (Il She Mu She)

One Begins Unmoved Moving, That Has No Beginning

一析三極無盡本 (Il Suk Sahm Guk Mu Jin Bohn)

One Divides To Three Crowns, While Remaining A Limitless Mover

天一一地一二人一三 (Chun Il Il Ji Il Ee In Il Sahm)

Heaven Comes First, Earth Comes Second, Human Comes Third

一積十鉅無匱化三 (Il Juk Ship Guh Mu Gweh Hwa Sahm)

One Gathers To Build Ten, And Infinite Forms Become The Trinity (of heaven, earth, human)

天二三地二三人二三 (Chun Ee Sahm Ji Ee Sahm In Ee Sahm)

Heaven Gains Two To Make Three, Earth Gains Two To Make Three, Human Gains Two To Make Three

大三合六生七八九運 (Dae Sahm Hahp Yook Saeng Chil Pahl Goo Une)
Three Trinities Make Six, And They Create Seven, And Eight, Nine
Appears, And There Comes A Turning

In looking at the cycle of creation and the evolution of life in terms of the numbers one through nine, the number six becomes a transition point. After going through six, life goes on to seven, eight, and nine, before going back to one. Everything, in its naturally ordained time, goes through deep renewal, a cosmic hibernation. Likewise, death is not really death. Once freed from the confines of the physical body, the soul evolves and assumes form in a higher dimension. Just as everything began with the One and will ultimately return to the One, the soul can be said to have completed its journey once it returns to where it came from.

The number six is also crucial in the human Chakra system. It refers not only to the 6th Chakra of our body, but also to the "六生 (Yook Saeng)" in the Heavenly Code, signifying "Birth of the Soul from the place of the 6th Chakra." If the 1st Chakra is the gate through which the body is born, then the 6th Chakra is the gate through which the soul is born. Once you have awakened to the birth of your soul, you are no longer fettered to the body, but can develop the "sight" to see life as an eternal force that exists in itself, of itself, and by itself.

The Principle of Su-Seung-Hwa-Gang
(Water Energy Up, Fire Energy Down)

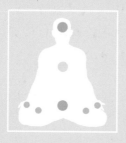

三四成環五七一 (Sahm Sah Sung Hwan Oh Chil Il)
Three And Four Form A Circle, Five With Seven Makes One Whole

妙衍萬汪萬來用變不動本
(Myo Yeon Mahn Wang Mahn Lae Yong Byun Bu Dong Bon)
Way-Less Is The Way All Comes And All Goes, Features Are Changing,
And Change-Less Is The Maker

Su-Seung-Hwa-Gang (Water Energy Up, Fire Energy Down)
refers to the direction in which energy must flow in the body in
order to create harmony and a healthy balance. Water energy must
travel up the meridian along the spine, while fire energy must travel
down the meridian along the centerline of the front of the body.
This is the optimal state of energy flow.

The "Three" in the first line above refers to the three main internal Chakras, the 2nd, the 4th, and the 6th. The "Four" in the first line above refers to the four external Chakras, located on each of the palms and the bottoms of both feet. The external Chakras located in the center of each palm are called "Jang-shim," and the external Chakras located in the center of each foot are called "Yong-chun." When the three major internal Chakras and the four external Chakras are working as one circle (Sung Hwan), the body is filled with free flowing, life-giving energy in accordance with the direction of Su-Seung-Hwa-Gang (Water Energy Up, Fire Energy Down).

The "Five, Seven, and One..." in the line above refer to the 5th, 7th, and 1st Chakras. When these Chakras, which are the three gates of life (to be explained later), are connected with the other four internal Chakras (2nd, 3rd, 4th, 6th), and with the four major external Chakras, the life force within us will flow freely, bringing infinite creativity and joy to the soul.

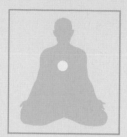

本心本太陽昂明 (Bon Shim Bon Tae Yang Ahng Myung)
Divine Mind Is Eternal Light, Looking Toward Celestial Light

"Bon Shim Bon" refers to the palace of the mind, the center. When the mind is at its proper center, then "Tae Yang Ahng Myung" occurs, which means that the mind becomes as bright as the sun. Mind is placed in the 4th Chakra. When the 4th Chakra is awakened and becomes bright, it shall awaken the 1st, 5th, and 7th Chakras, thereby attaining freedom of the soul. Someone who has attained true freedom of the soul is called "Shin In," or Divine Person.

When the soul attains true freedom, it escapes the limitations of the body, without life or death, beginning or end, and reaches the place of the One. Healing Chakra is, therefore, based on the principle of activating the Chakra system for the purpose of enlightening divinity within for completion of the soul's journey.

20

The Principle of the Oneness of the Cosmic Self

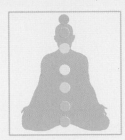

人中天地一 (In Joong Chun Ji Il)

Human Bears Heaven And Earth, And The Three Make One

"Human Bears Heaven and Earth," refers to the person who has realized the Self as part of the Grand Oneness of the Cosmos. Such a person is also a "Shin In," or divine person. Healing Chakra is a training system designed to allow one to experience the Self as part of the whole cosmos. When all seven internal Chakras are awakened, or activated, you will realize Oneness with the rest of the cosmos, knowing that Heaven and Earth are within you.

The Principle of Eternal Life

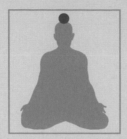

一終無終一 (Il Jong Mu Jong Il)
One Is The End Of All, And The One Has No Ending

The physical body has a beginning and an end. However, the soul is timeless and limitless. Knowing this, you are liberated from fear, attaining true peace of mind, freedom of imagination, and infinite creativity of the spirit. When the soul leaves a person's body through the 7th Chakra, that individual is said to have undergone a Heavenly Transformation.

3. The Chakras and the Process of Completing the Soul

There are three gates and three palaces, which we must pass through in order to attain completion of the soul. Awakening the Chakras, by ascending the Chakra ladder, will lead you to the third human birth, the spiritual birth of Heavenly Transformation.

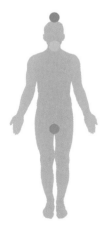

Three Gates

Jade Gate (Ok Muhn):
Signifies the 1st Chakra, located at the perineum point. It is the gate through which the seed of life enters. It is also the gate through which the body is born. Life's first birth, the birth of the body, occurs through the Jade Gate.

Soul Gate (Hohn Muhn):
Signifies the 5th Chakra, located around the thyroid glands in the

neck. Most of our souls are trapped in the physical body. In order for a soul to be born through the 6th Chakra, it must escape the 4th and pass through the 5th Chakra. When the Soul Gate opens, the seed of the soul enters the palace of the 6th Chakra to begin growing. Once you pass through the Soul Gate, you will feel a true sense of freedom. You will no longer be deceived by the cycle of highs and lows based on material gain and external circumstances. When you attain true freedom of the soul, frustration and emptiness will disappear naturally.

Heaven's Gate (Chun Muhn):
Also called the Great Heaven's Gate (Dae Chun Muhn), this refers to the 7th Chakra, located around the Baek-hwe point. Its literal meaning is "Gate that connects to Heaven." In Asia, it was much revered. Just as the body gestates in the womb and is born through the Jade Gate, the soul gestates in the palace of the 6th Chakra and is born through Heaven's Gate. This is the birth of the Spiritual Body.

Three Palaces

Earth Palace (Ji or Jah Goong):
Refers to the 2nd Chakra, located in the lower Dahn-jon. This is the place where sperm and ovum meet to create and nurture the body. It is often referred to as the Earth Palace because it is the place where the body is prepared for birth into life on Earth.

Mind Palace (Shim Goong):
Refers to the 4th Chakra, where the middle Dahn-jon is located. It is referred to as the Mind Palace, because it is believed to house the mind. It is also the place of emotions, including loneliness, sadness, and love. Someone who is full of compassion and love is often referred to as a "humane" person. The 4th Chakra is termed the "Human Palace" (In Goong). In order to open Heaven's Gate, all of the Chakras from the 1st through the 7th must be connected. The 4th Chakra is especially important in this connection. You must open your mind and rid yourself of attachment and greed in order to awaken the 4th Chakra.

Heaven's Palace
Refers to the 6th Chakra, where the upper Dahn-jon, or In-dang is located. This is the place where the soul dwells with the presence of heaven. When the soul passes through the Soul's Gate (5th Chakra) and enters into Heaven's Palace, it begins to mature, readying itself for a spiritual birth through Heaven's Gate (7th Chakra).

The Three Births

Human beings have the potential to undergo three separate births. First is the physical birth, in which the body is born through the Jade Gate of the 1st Chakra. Second is the awakening, in which you realize that the essence of your being is your soul. This awakening occurs in the 6th Chakra. The third birth refers to the birth of the spiritual body through Heaven's Gate, the 7th Chakra. When you have achieved the third birth, you will have attained Oneness with the cosmos, completion of the soul.

The body is akin to a vehicle driven by the soul. The body must be left behind in order for the soul to be born through Heaven's Gate. The analogy is rather simple. In order for you to enter the house, you have to get out of your vehicle. You only need the car to get you to your house. In order for your soul to be born through Heaven's Gate, it must mature and become complete. The picture of a small baby on top of the head in the Chakra drawing refers to this spiritual birth... a Heavenly Transformation.

In the tradition of Shin-Sun-Do, the process of the completion and birth of the soul is called "Sung Tong Gong Wan." "Sung Tong" refers to awakening, or enlightenment. "Gong Wan" refers to the real effort and work required for a person to actualize enlightenment in the real world. Therefore, the process involves both profound internal awakening and real effort to actualize this new awareness in the world.

Healing Chakra of the Soul

Do you remember your immediate past? I am not asking you to recall your previous lives, but rather to think about your recent past in this life... on a biological level. This may be a trick question of sorts, but no less true because of it.

You were a sperm. And you were an ovum. Then, you were an embryo and a fetus. Then, you were a baby, born into this world with the body of a human being. Some of you were received warmly, while others of you were not. This is not too important in the overall scheme of things.

Do you know the odds of being born as a human being, not in a metaphysical sense, but in a biological sense? In the Buddhist tradition, they say the odds of being born as a human being are the same odds as a sea turtle encountering a wooden plank floating in the middle of the Pacific Ocean as it comes up for air. Let's examine the odds in a biological sense. We all know how a baby is conceived. With each ejaculation, between 100 and 150 million sperm are released. Of those, only one gets to impregnate the ovum, resulting in conception. So, the odds of conception are about 1 in 100 million. However, the odds are actually even higher than this, since not every sexual encounter will result in either ejaculation or the introduction of sperm into the vagina. Frankly, calculating all the social factors that go into a couple's decision to bear a child, the odds of a human being as unique as you being born is truly unimaginable. The odds are literally astronomical. Being born as a human being is akin to a roll of the cosmic dice. That is why birth as a human being is a great blessing, too great to truly articulate.

But, what is the purpose of being born as a human being? To attain the physical body? No. You already know what it is... The purpose of a human birth is to complete the journey of your soul, to manifest your essence as a spiritual being, to effect the birth of your spiritual body. This is also the purpose of the Chakra system and Healing Chakra.

So, how do we achieve this completion? Let's skip the amorphous, esoteric, and new age jargon that passes for spirituality these days. Instead, we can explain the process of spiritual birth using the Chakra system. We can think about this process of spiritual birth as part of our natural anatomy. To initiate the process of our physical birth, the sperm enters through the Jade Gate, the first Chakra, and lodges in the Earth Palace or Womb, the second Chakra. A life is conceived when the sperm joins with an ovum. After nine months of gestation, the physical body matures and is born, once again passing through the Jade Gate. These are the fundamentals of our reproductive system.

Now, let's think about the spiritual birth process. The sperm is analogous to the seed of the soul, while the ovum is analogous to the divinity within us. The spiritual sperm, or seed of the soul, is not some abstract concept, however. It resides in the heart, the fourth Chakra, intertwined with the presence of energy there. Then where does the spiritual ovum reside? It lives in the sixth Chakra, which is also called Heaven's Palace. Therefore, the process of spiritual birth is ignited when the spiritual sperm and the spiritual ovum merge in Heaven's Palace, the spiritual womb within the human body. In order for the merging to take effect, the spiritual sperm, like the physical sperm, must pass through a gate. This gate is the fifth Chakra, or the Soul's Gate. When the seed of the soul passes through the Soul's Gate and lodges in Heaven's Palace, where it meets with inner divinity, a spiritual embryo is conceived. After a process of maturation and growth, the spiritual body is born

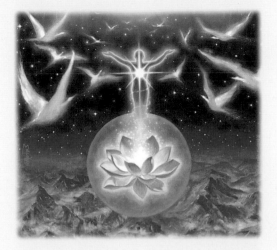

through the seventh Chakra, also called the Great Heaven's Gate.

Now you understand the meaning behind the terms that we use to denote the individual Chakras. It is this process of spiritual birth that differentiates us from other animals. It is why human beings are spiritual beings. Therefore, as a human being, you have an incredible opportunity to express your spiritual essence in a profound way. Once your spiritual body is born, you are ready to merge with Cosmic Energy and Cosmic Mind, the essence of the Creator. You are a child of the Creator, holding the seed of the Creator Within. You are the sons and daughters of God.

The Chakra system serves as the reservoir of the spiritual potential within us. If our physical body is our temple, then our energy body, as represented by the Chakra system, is our altar upon which we will stand and rise to our rightful place as a spiritual being, in tune with the great truth and cycle of the cosmos. To achieve this is our ultimate goal in life. Healing Chakra is our way of beginning this journey of the soul.

Change Your Energy

Change Your Brain

Change Your Life

Part II
Energy and Our Body

1. Three Different Types of Bodies

How can the often-abstract concept of 'Inner Divinity' or 'Completion of the Soul' be easily explained and experienced in today's world? The answer lies with energy. Healing Chakra is a training regimen that focuses on the energy centers of the body. Called "Ki" in Asian tradition, this energy acts as a bridge that connects the body to the soul.

In order to understand the Chakra system of the body, we must first understand the structure of the energy system that sustains life. We have three different bodies. The first is the physical body, which we can see and touch. Most of us think that this is all there is to being human.

We also have an energy body. If you have developed sensitivity to energy, you can sense a soft sheath of energy encapsulating your body. Chakras are energy centers, which are part of the energy body. Within the energy body, there are specific places where energy gathers. These points are called Dahn-jons. We have three internal Dahn-jons that correspond to the 2nd, 4th, and 6th Chakras. There are also four external Dahn-jons: one in the center of each our palms and one in the center of the upper third of the sole of each foot. Together with the three internal Dahn-jons, this constitutes the seven Chakra system.

Finally, we have a spiritual body. It surrounds both the physical and energy bodies and is the master of both. These three bodies form an organic relationship, influencing our physical, mental, and emotional health.

The energy body acts as a bridge connecting our physical and spiritual bodies. In order for us to influence, or effect a transformation of the body and mind, we must first learn to transform the

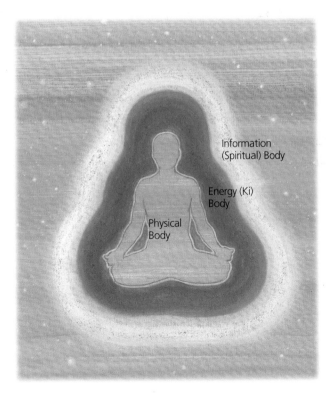

Information (Spiritual) Body

Energy (Ki) Body

Physical Body

energy flow. The essence of Healing Chakra and Heavenly Transformation is the use of energy to effect the completion of the soul. Without knowing energy, you cannot approach your soul.

An imbalance in the energy body originates from spiritual problems. You can affect the state of the energy body with your thoughts and state of mind. If your mind receives negative information, or generates negative emotions, it will influence your energy body accordingly. We often think that physical diseases have only physical causes, however, before a disease or illness is physically manifested, it can be predicted by a pattern of energy imbalance.

2. Chakras and the Brain

It is common knowledge that we utilize only ten percent of the full capacity of the human brain. All of humankind's achievements in the areas of art, music, science, literature, as well as all works of genius, have resulted from use of a mere ten percent of the human brain. Utilization of the brain means that we become conscious of the latent potential in areas of the brain that we are not currently using. The way to wake up the brain is to infuse the entire brain with energy while expanding consciousness to include every area. Awakening the brain is a matter of expanding consciousness.

The seven Chakras of the body are directly related to different areas of the brain. By analogy: if Ki energy is equivalent to electricity, and the Chakras are the switches, then each area of the brain is a light. Just as you turn a light on by activating a switch, you can awaken the parts of the brain by activating the Chakras. If only one Chakra is turned on, then only the part of the brain corresponding to that Chakra will awaken. And in order for a human being to become one with the divine spirituality within, the whole brain must be awakened.

Chakras also have a direct symbiotic relationship with the autonomic nervous system. This is the system that controls the most basic life functions of respiration, circulation, and digestion. The Chakras also have an intimate relationship with the endocrine system. Blockages or imbalances in the energy of the Chakras are reflected in the types and levels of hormones released by the endocrine system.

Conversely, pain or problems in a particular area of the physical body are transmitted to the corresponding Chakra. For example,

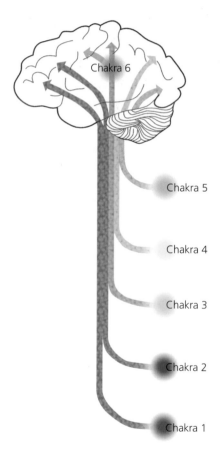

Activating The Chakras As They Relate To The Brain

Chakras may be activated one by one, or as a whole system. However, each Chakra, once activated, will stimulate the associated center of the brain through the energy connection and will allow the user to undergo an experience that is unique to the said center of the brain. For example, activating the second Chakra will stimulate the brain to generate a joyful emotion. Activating the third Chakra will generate a strong sense of the self. Fourth will produce love, while fifth will generate the ability to judge or evaluate. Sixth will result in an enhancement of intuition and supernormal sensitivity.

the sexual organs are connected to the 1st Chakra, the reproductive and excretory organs and functions are connected to the 2nd Chakra, and so forth...

Until now, the collective human consciousness has generally remained at the level of the 1st, 2nd, and 3rd Chakras. Sexual appetite, fear, anxiety, desire, and despair are manifested when consciousness is trapped at the level of the lower three Chakras. We currently live in a society obsessed with sex, money, and other physical and material desires. Full activation of the Chakra system is not only an important matter for the individual, but for all of human society as well. For when we activate the 4th through the 7th Chakras, and utilize their connection to the profound energies of the universe, we will stimulate and thus awaken higher planes of human existence, consisting of wisdom, love, mercy, and insight, among others.

The three layers of the human brain and Chakras

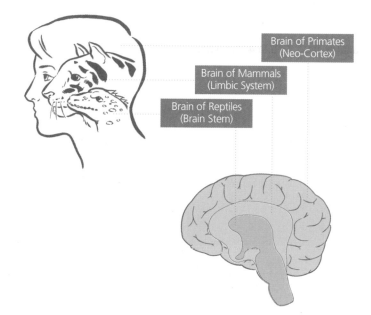

Brain of Primates
(Neo-Cortex)

Brain of Mammals
(Limbic System)

Brain of Reptiles
(Brain Stem)

The human brain can be divided into three layers, with each layer corresponding to each evolutionary stage. The reptilian brain is simple, geared only to the maintenance of survival functions: respiration, digestion, circulation, and reproduction. Extending out of the reptilian brain is the mammalian brain, adding the capacity for emotion and coordination of movement. The third phase of evolution resulted in the cerebral cortex, which provides the ability to solve problems, be creative, and develop memory - the cerebral cortex can be called the human Brain.

Reptilian Brain - 1ST and 2ND Chakras

The brain stem consists of various sub-cortical structures. It maintains basic survival functions, including respiration, digestion, circulation, and reproduction. It corresponds to humans' deepest subconscious, often becoming the major driving force behind life. Most people spend their time satisfying the needs of the 1ST and 2ND Chakras, which includes satisfying the need for food, shelter, and sexual release.

Mammalian Brain - 3RD and 4TH Chakras

Corresponds to the limbic system of the brain - or the evolutionary second layer. Controls emotions such as joy, sadness, excitement, surprise, amazement, and love, among others. A problem with the limbic layer will create abnormal emotional responses. The limbic system also controls anger, fear, guilt, worry, pain, joy... and a range of other human emotional responses.

Human Brain - 5TH and 6TH Chakras

Corresponds to the Cerebral Cortex or the Neo-Cortex, which enables us to create and introspect. Of these, the frontal lobe is the latest creation, giving us the ability to think and speculate. The ability of the Neo-Cortex to have insight, think, and rationalize helps to activate the 5TH and 6TH Chakras. Therefore, a frontal lobotomy will often result in lack of imagination and interest in life. The Neo-Cortex is the mastermind behind all the glory of the human culture and civilization that we have created.

3. Light, Sound, and Vibration

Chakras are awakened and activated through energy. Energy exists in three forms: light, sound, and vibration. These three forms are basic to the creation of the universe. This is expressed by the word Yullyo. All of life exists within Yullyo. Healing Chakra seeks to create balanced energy flow to stimulate and awaken the sense of Yullyo within all of us.

Yullyo resides in Heaven's Palace, corresponding to the 6th Chakra, which is in turn directly connected to the brain stem. The brain stem is the gate through which Yullyo manifests. It is literally the seat of inner divinity.

Vibration is the quickest way to approach and stimulate the brain stem, which controls all basic life functions. Chakra activation begins with stimulation of the brain stem. Vibration is the essence of all of life's activities. All life, including each cell of our bodies, has a frequency of vibration. From the tiniest grain of sand to the largest of stars, all matter has a unique, characteristic frequency. It is the grand vibration of the cosmos that forms the essence of the grand harmony of the universe, within which chaos, creation, and evolution are generated.

Light, sound, and vibration exist within our bodies. Each of our internal organs has its characteristic and unique sound. Just as the heart beats, the brain, liver, stomach, kidneys, and other organs have their respective voices, which combined form a beautiful symphony.

Through vibration, our bodies continuously shed old cells and create new ones. This is a normal life process. By utilizing the natural healing power within all of us, persons with a healthy vibration can heal themselves, even when confronted with injury or illness. If a particular organ has a problem, it begins to emit a discordant tone. The rest of the body's organs then generate a harmonious, healing symphony, in an attempt to resolve the problem by helping the compromised organ regain its proper frequency. However, once the body's harmonious voice is weakened or broken, its healing power is compromised. Thus, illness can manifest. Negative thoughts and a negative mind are the primary cause of the breakdown, leading to discordant notes among the body's organs.

Healing Chakra is designed to help each person recognize the naturally occurring frequency of vibration within. And further... to discover that it is a part of the overall symphony of the universe!

Change Your Energy

Change Your Brain

Change Your Life

Part Ⅲ
Healing Chakra Exercises

Within the Energy

Lie the Secrets to Healing Body, Mind, and Soul

Transformation of the Energy

Changes Habits, Personality, Body, and Thoughts

1. Chakra Relaxation

Before beginning Healing Chakra Training, it is important to relax your body and mind. Unless you are sensitive to Ki energy, you cannot activate your body's Chakra system. Ki energy is felt when body and mind are in a relaxed state. Relaxation is prerequisite to all forms of meditation and healing. When we are tense, our minds and bodies tend to contract, thus prohibiting the free flow of energy.

Ki energy acts as a bridge connecting body and soul. The soul delivers its messages to the body through Ki energy. You must relax in order to meet with your soul. Ji-gam (energy sensitivity training) and Dahn-mu (energy dance) are the most effective methods to induce relaxation. Ji-gam training assists in stopping the flow of thoughts and emotions, making it possible to concentrate exclusively on the body. With this heightened sensitivity, it is possible to expand the feeling of the subtle currents of energy. As your state of Ji-gam becomes deeper, your body will move with the flow of energy in an unconscious, spontaneous expression of the energy flow. This is Dahn-mu. Through Dahn-mu, you will meet with your true master, your soul. Thus, Dahn-mu is the language of the soul.

Through Ki energy, you can communicate with any organ of your body. Ki energy is omnipresent, not only within our bodies, but throughout the universe. Ki goes where our mind directs it. If we consciously think about our heart and brain, Ki will flow there. Dahn-mu is a way of expressing currents of energy with your movements. The moment you immerse yourself in the currents of energy, beyond the barriers of self-consciousness and thought, you begin to converse with your soul. This is the moment when the divinity within awakens. "My body is not my all." "My emotions are not my all." "My thoughts are not my all."

"Then, what or who am I?" "Who is the real me?" Only through Ki energy can you meet with your True Self. Dahn-mu is a signal that you are ready to meet the Creator Within. To feel the flow of Ki energy, and to use it to awaken the deepest potential within, is truly a blessing and will bring about transformation of your life.

Self-Observation

Sit or stand in a comfortable position
And close your eyes.
Before meeting with your soul,
Let us take this opportunity to meet with the body.
In order to meet with your body,
You must separate your consciousness
From your body.
Whisper to yourself...

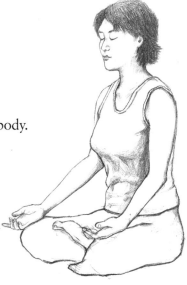

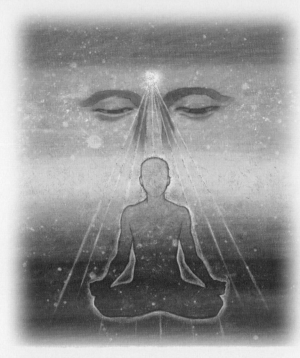

My body is not me, but mine.
My mouth is not me, but mine.
My head is not me, but mine.
My eyes are not me, but mine.
My legs are not me, but mine.
My arms are not me, but mine.
My chest is not me, but mine.
My thoughts are not me, but mine.
My emotions are not me, but mine.

Whisper to yourself continuously,
As you feel every part of your body,
From your head to your toes...
Whisper to yourself

With confidence and conviction
Until you feel yourself looking at your body.
Who is the master of my body?
My soul is the master of my body.

Raise your hands slowly in front of your chest.
Then let your hands go where they will,
Legs, arms, chest...
You are holding a private conversation with your body.
Now bring your hands together, on your chest
And speak to your soul...
Bringing mind and body together...

Ji-gam (Energy Sensitivity) Training

Raise both hands to chest level,
Palms facing each other, but not touching...
Direct your consciousness to your hands
And whisper, "Hands...hands...hands..."
With the voice of your mind.
Feel your hands begin to react.
A certain pull, a warmth...
Something drifting between your hands...
You are feeling the sensation of energy.
Now push your hands closer together.

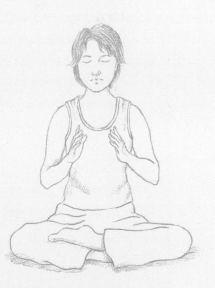

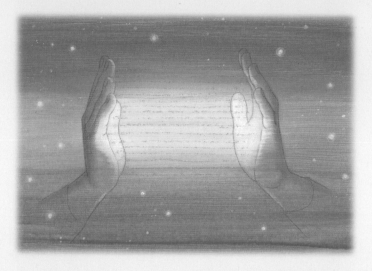

When you think, "My hands are coming closer together..."
Then they will draw closer.
When you think, "My hands are moving farther apart..."
Then they will move away from each other.
You can control your hands with your mind.
Repeat the pull-push motions,
Affirming the sensation of energy between your hands.

Now, imagine a ball of energy between your hands.
Pour your consciousness into the space between your hands.
Feel the cloud of energy, tangible and alive.
Expand on the living sensation,
Molding it into the shape of a ball.
Smooth the edges until it becomes a sphere...
A ball full of air and bounce.

You have just created a ball of energy with your hands.
Such is the way of energy and your mind.
This is the energy that will free the energies of your Chakras.

When you concentrate on a certain part of your body,
Blood flows to that part, energy gathers, and heat generates.
A pulse beats and a magnetic energy exists.
Consciousness communicates with the brain.
The brain sends blood where you will it to go,
And energy follows.

This is a way of training the brain.
This is the way to awaken the brain.
The brain moves only by the energy.

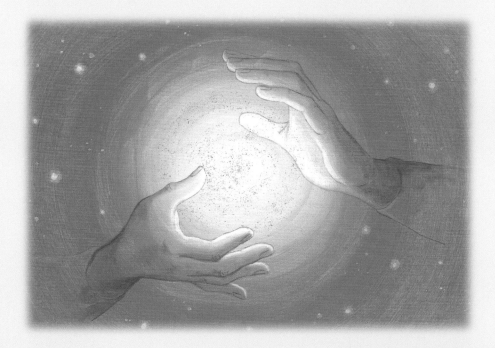

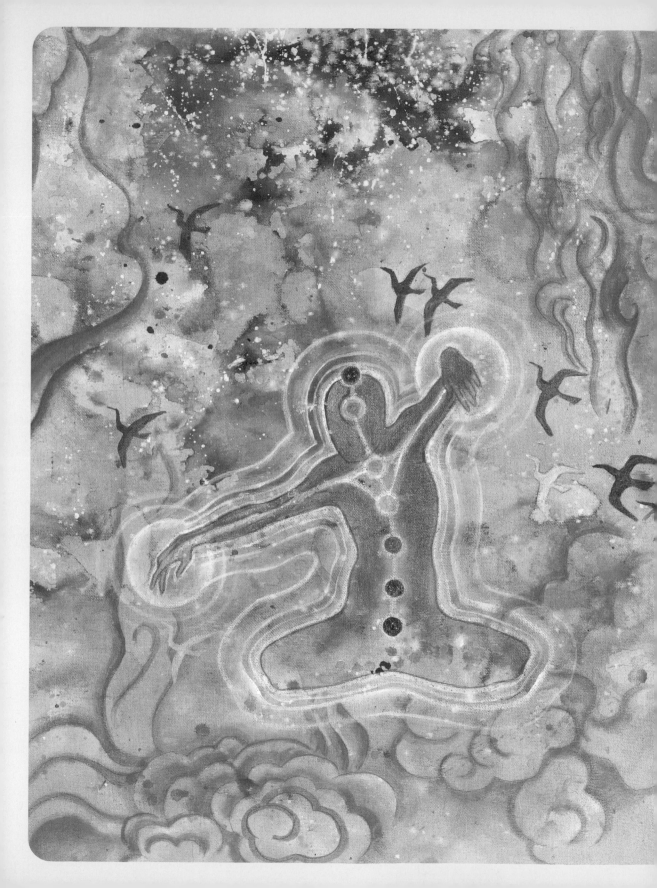

Dahn-mu

Relax your arms and let them fall to your sides.
Let the currents of energy take you where they will...
Let go of logic and rational thought.
Let exuberance and spontaneity take over...
You no longer feel any weight in your hands.
They are floating freely in the gentle current of
The great sea of energy.
Your hands, your neck, your shoulders... all are moving freely.
Your arms, legs, and waist... all dance without gravity.
You are spontaneous with your exuberance.
And exuberant at your spontaneity...
Free... so free... This is Dahn-mu.

Until now, your left-brain ruled the day.
Logical, rational, and strict...
A prison of negative information and memory...
Now, rest your left-brain and give your right-brain free rein.
For your right brain knows what you need.
Let the right brain move you in all the right ways...
In all the right places...
To fill you with passion, love, and peace...
And clear your tangled thoughts and emotions.
Feel the Chakras move and stir...
And your soul call out for freedom.

Hold a conversation with your soul
As you dance the Dance of Energy.
Dahn-mu will move you with the flow of energy.

It is unlike any way you have ever moved,
Unlike any dance you have ever danced.
Thoughts move your body through nerves,
As the soul moves your body through Ki.
Within Ki your soul breathes...
When you feel Ki energy,
You are experiencing your soul.
You are relaxed... purified.

2. Feeling Your Chakras

Locating the Chakras in Your Body

"Nae Gwan," directly translated, means "inner watching." Through Nae Gwan, you use the eye of your mind to look deeply into your body. You begin to awaken and activate the Chakras through deep relaxation and concentration. The law of energy movement, Shim-Ki-Hyul-Jung states: "Where mind goes, energy follows; where energy goes, blood follows; where blood goes, strength follows." Accordingly, we can activate the Chakras by concentrating with our mind. Let us explore the sensation of each individual Chakra.

At first, due to unfamiliarity, it is difficult to feel the exact location of the Chakras within your body. The first step in the process is to identify the location of each Chakra and to focus on the feeling until you become familiar with its sensation. After a while, with concentration, you will quickly be able to locate the sensation of the individual Chakras.

As seen in the diagram, the Chakras are located roughly along the line of your spine. Because Chakras are energy centers, they do not necessarily correspond to specific anatomical locations. Since the Chakras are energy, they are not visible, like blood and bones. Therefore, it is easier to try to imagine the exact location of each Chakra by locating its corresponding point on the front of the body. By identifying general physical landmarks on the front of the body, it will be possible to communicate the location of specific Chakras on which to concentrate.

The first and seventh Chakras do not have corresponding points on the front of the body. However, the second Chakra corresponds to the lower Dahn-jon, the third Chakra to the Joong-wahn point, located two inches above the navel, the fourth Chakra to the Dahn-joong, located at the sternum, and the fifth Chakra to the front of the thyroid glands. The sixth Chakra corresponds to the proverbial "third eye" on your forehead.

From the first through the seventh Chakra, we will touch upon the sensation of each individual Chakra.

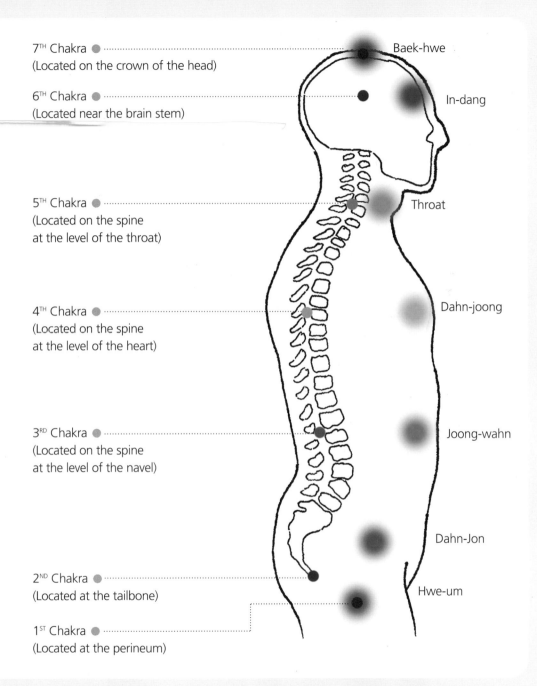

7TH Chakra ●
(Located on the crown of the head)

6TH Chakra ●
(Located near the brain stem)

5TH Chakra ●
(Located on the spine
at the level of the throat)

4TH Chakra ●
(Located on the spine
at the level of the heart)

3RD Chakra ●
(Located on the spine
at the level of the navel)

2ND Chakra ●
(Located at the tailbone)

1ST Chakra ●
(Located at the perineum)

Baek-hwe

In-dang

Throat

Dahn-joong

Joong-wahn

Dahn-Jon

Hwe-um

▲ Locations of the Chakra, along the line of your spine, and their corresponding
energy points along the front surface of the body. These energy points and physical landmarks will help in feeling and visualizing each Chakra.

First Chakra - Hwe-um

Sit in half lotus position with your back straight.
Concentrate on the first Chakra.
For men concentrate on your Hwe-um, between the anus and base of the penis.
For women, concentrate on the back of the uterus
Between the urethra and anus.
If you can't feel the area,
Contract and relax your sphincter muscle repeatedly.
As you repeat this exercise,
Imagine a stream of breath coming in and out of the first Chakra.
Men should concentrate on the feeling of pressure on the Hwe-um.
Women should concentrate on the feeling near the opening of the uterus,
Which is located about one inch below the end of the spine.
Through repeated contraction/relaxation of the sphincter muscle,
You can awaken the sensation of the first Chakra,
Amplifying the energy in the area.
Repeat the contraction/relaxation 100 times.
You will have a sensation of heat,
As energy courses through your body.
A healthy first Chakra is the color of clear red,
Imparting a feeling of warmth.
A problematic first Chakra turns to the color of a dying ember.

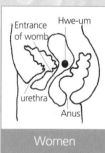

Entrance of womb — Hwe-um — urethra — Anus

Women

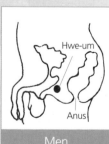

Hwe-um — Anus

Men

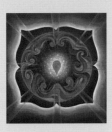

Source of All Energy

A four-leaf lotus flower with a deep red color represents the first Chakra. This Chakra is the place where the body meets the earth. It is the place where energy flows into the body. When this Chakra is weak, energy can also be lost through this area. The first Chakra is the source of all creation and growth, undulating with the pure energy of life. The first Chakra must be fully functional in order to activate the other Chakras. It acts as a pump that helps the stream of energy rise along the spine. This imparts a sense of confidence and a love of life, creating a positive energy field that influences others.

A person with a healthy first Chakra is full of life and the will to grow. If your first Chakra is blocked or impeded, you will experience a lack of will, vigor, and passion. Without sufficient physical energy, the body cannot act as a solid anchor for consciousness, resulting in the lack of a sense of reality. This may result in the appearance of illness and oversensitivity to external circumstances. Spiritual richness can only arise with plenty of energy.

Second Chakra - Dahn-jon

The second Chakra is located at the very end of the tailbone.
In order to activate the second Chakra,
Concentrate on your lower Dahn-jon,
Which is located about two inches below your navel.
The second Chakra connects to the prostate gland in men.
In women, it is connected to the uterus.
It is also connected to the reproductive organs, bladder, and kidneys.
When you breathe in, imagine a stream of air entering your body
Through the 'Myung-moon' point in your lower back,
Curling and swirling as it enters...
When you breathe out, imagine the stream of air uncurling as it exits.
When you breathe in, your lower abdomen expands
When you breathe out... your lower abdomen contracts...
Continue breathing as you are feeling your Dahn-jon,
The second Chakra.
You may feel emptiness in your lower Dahn-jon,
You may experience a feeling of fullness...
Silently follow the path of your breath.
You will feel warmth in your Dahn-jon.
You may feel a beating pulse coming alive.

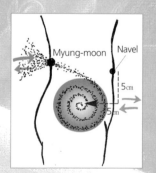

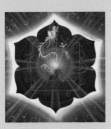

Creative and Sexual Energy

The symbol of the second Chakra is a six-leaf, scarlet lotus flower. Along with the first Chakra, the second Chakra controls sexual energy. A person with a healthy second Chakra has strength, while a person with a blocked second Chakra easily feels fatigued.

The lower Dahn-jon is where the earth's energy, flowing in through the 'Yong-chun' points, combines with both the energy of heaven, coming in as you breathe, and the energy of life that exists within us all. Here these energies merge and are transformed into a higher form of energy.

Energies gathered in the lower Dahn-jon also stimulate the kidneys to elevate water energy and lower fire energy, facilitating optimal flow of energy according to the Law of Su-Seung-Hwa-Gang (Water Energy Up, Fire Energy Down). This results in a relaxed mind, clear head, and strong Dahn-jon.

The second Chakra mounts a defense system around the body to protect it from toxins in foodstuff, nervous disorders, and contagious diseases. It cleanses the body of deeply rooted tension and stress that inhibit procreative activities.

Activation of the second Chakra also translates into maternal love and charity for others, resulting in harmonious relationships characterized by forgiveness and comfort. However, a blocked or impaired second Chakra may lead to negativity and jealousy, resulting in miscommunication with others. It may also lead to maternal love based on control and domination.

Third Chakra - Joong-wahn

The third Chakra is located straight behind the navel.
When you concentrate,
Concentrate on the spot two inches above your navel.
Using your fingers,
Press on the point two inches above your navel,
On the point called the Joong-wahn.
Now release the pressure of your fingers.
Concentrate on the point just behind them.
Feel the beating of your pulse.
When you inhale,
Breath comes in through the Joong-wahn point.
When you exhale, the breath goes out the same way.
Observe the organs surrounding the Joong-wahn
With your mind's eye...
The third Chakra connects with the stomach.
It also controls the liver, gall bladder and pancreas.

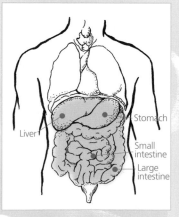

Liver
Stomach
Small intestine
Large intestine

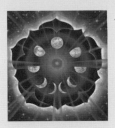

Physical Digestion and Metabolism

A ten-leaf, orange lotus flower symbolizes the third Chakra. A healthy third Chakra is bright orange, while a weak or blocked one may be a whitish or even bluish color. The third Chakra controls the body's metabolism and overall functioning. It is the seat of the physical self. An active and healthy third Chakra generates enthusiasm and passion for work. When the third Chakra is operating properly and harmoniously, rich emotions are present. A weakened third Chakra allows increased emotional vulnerability.

The third Chakra relates to the element of fire and is located on the spot called the "Tae Yang" nerve center in Oriental Medicine. It controls ambition and appetite, facilitating balanced metabolism. You can easily tell the state of your third Chakra by observing your appetite. When the third Chakra is weak, you will have a decreased appetite for food. Excessive appetite is also indicative of a Chakra that is unbalanced.

The third Chakra also connects with the neo-cortex. Accordingly, it is very sensitive to stress. If stress is prolonged, deterioration of the internal organs will occur. It is important to maintain a calm and peaceful state of mind in order to maximize efficiency of the third Chakra and the internal organs.

Fourth Chakra - Dahn-joong

The fourth Chakra is located behind the heart,
Toward the back and middle of the chest.
When you concentrate,
Concentrate on your Dahn-joong
Marked by the slight indentation on your chest, or sternum...
Using your fingers, press on your Dahn-joong.
Now release the pressure of your fingers.
Concentrate on the point just behind the pressure.
Breathe in slowly and let your chest expand.
Breathe out and let your chest contract.
Breathe in... and breathe out...
Imagine the breath streaming in and out of your Dahn-joong.
Concentrate on the fourth Chakra,
And expand the sensation.
You are feeling the source of energy for love and devotion.
Gently probe the state of your heart.
Do you feel blocked or open, comfortable or stuffy?
When the fourth Chakra is weak,
The 'Im Maek,' a major meridian running through the chest,
Becomes blocked.

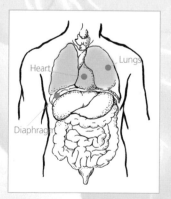

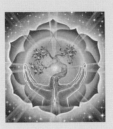

Our Humanness

A twelve-leaf, golden lotus flower symbolizes the fourth Chakra. The fourth Chakra expands our energy and sends it in all directions in equal parts. It also acts to harmonize opposing energies, such as male/female, yin/yang, and emotional/logical. The fourth Chakra is located right in the center of the Chakra ladder. There are three chakras above it, and three below. When the fourth Chakra, which links the energies of body and mind together, becomes active, you experience a sense of pure love and compassion. This arises out of a balance of mind and body.

The fourth Chakra relates to the human attributes of love, forgiveness, honesty, responsibility, and diligence. A healthy fourth Chakra creates a balanced and harmonious energy of love. It facilitates the balance of logic with emotion, and the real with the ideal, helping you to develop the maturity to be objective and unconditional in your love of others. You will give and receive love from a centered and balanced place.

Fifth Chakra - Throat

The fifth Chakra is located just behind your throat, by the thyroid glands.
Lightly press down on your throat,
On the spot where a man's Adams apple is located.
Now, release the pressure of your fingers.
Concentrate on the point just behind where the pressure was.
Lightly touch the roof of your mouth with your tongue.
Breathe in, as you imagine a stream of breath enter the fifth Chakra.
Breathe out as you imagine a stream of breath
Leaving through the same spot...
Breathe in as you bend your head backward...
Breathe out as you come back up.
Breathe in as you bend your head forward...
Breathe out as you come back up.
Rotate your head from side to side.

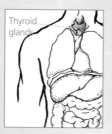

Thyroid glands

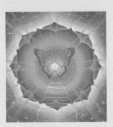

Energy of Purification and Harmony

A sixteen-leaf lotus flower is the symbol of the fifth Chakra. It is a blue-green color, with a tinge of yellow. The fifth Chakra is the center for purification and cleansing. This Chakra represents an open heart and mind. An open mind leads to a greater understanding of life. A person with an open mind goes through life embracing discomfort along with comfort, the bad along with the good... the vinegar with the wine. Such a person possesses the wisdom to go along with the flow of life.

A problem with the fifth Chakra translates into a lack of emotional control and rapid fatigue arising out of hypersensitivity to change. This Chakra is the bridge between aspects of the animal-human and the spiritual-human. It determines whether you live a more animalistic or a more spiritual life.

This is why we refer to the fifth Chakra as the Soul's Gate. Without going through this gate, you cannot move into the realm of the spiritually divine. With the fifth Chakra closed, emptiness of spirit drives an attempt to attain lasting fulfillment with riches and recognition. This emptiness is a message from your soul. We can experience true peace only when we go through the Soul's Gate of the fifth Chakra. Without pure consciousness and mind, it will be impossible to open its doors.

Sixth Chakra - In-dang

The sixth Chakra is located in the brain stem.
It is directly connected to the "In-dang" point between the eyebrows.
Lightly press down on that center point,
A half an inch above your eyebrows...
Now release the pressure of your fingers.
Concentrate on the point just behind them.
While feeling the beating of your pulse through the In-dang,
Maintain the sensation of pressure.
Lifting both hands,
Press down and massage the temples on both sides of your head.
Now release the pressure.
Imagine a thin line of energy that connects the two temple points.
Now draw a line from the center of the temple line
To your In-dang.
Form a T-line of energy inside your head.
Concentrate on the point of intersection
Where it bisects the brain stem...
Breathe in and feel the breath enter the In-dang.
Breathe out and feel the breath exit through the In-dang.

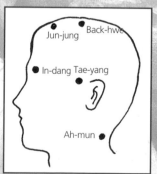

Jun-jung Back-hwe

In-dang Tae-yang

Ah-mun

66

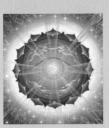

Awakening the Soul

A dark blue lotus flower represents the sixth Chakra. The role of the sixth Chakra is to combine energy from the lower five Chakras and elevate it to a higher plane. The energy of the sixth Chakra transcends time, integrating past, present, and future into a single moment, the "eternal now." This is why we refer to it as "The Third Eye." When the sixth Chakra is open, one may have insight into the nature of time and the universe, heightened instinct, superior insight, and the ability to give tangible form to imagination.

One with an active and functional sixth Chakra immediately sees into the heart of a problem, offering help where it is needed most. With a finger on the pulse of the future, this person will be able to navigate wisely through the present. On the other hand, someone with a weak sixth Chakra lacks a flow of fresh, creative ideas and cannot easily translate ideas into reality.

One often experiences special abilities when the sixth Chakra is active. Just as physical life begins with conception in the womb, spiritual life begins with spiritual conception in the sixth Chakra. When the soul awakens, a human can feel genuine love, mercy, and compassion for the earth and her creatures.

Seventh Chakra - Baek-hwe

Shift your awareness to the Baek-hwe point
On top of your head... the seventh Chakra.
As the sixth Chakra awakens,
The seventh Chakra follows.
Maintaining the energy lines from the sixth Chakra,
Connect them to the Baek-hwe point.
Lightly press down on the crown of your head.
Now release the pressure of your fingers.
Expand the sensation of the Chakra.
Feel the vibration that radiates outward
From the In-dang to the Baek-hwe
In-dang... Baek-hwe...
Now imagine a swirling vortex of energy
Being drawn into the Baek-hwe...
A solid pillar of energy
Connecting all of your Chakras...

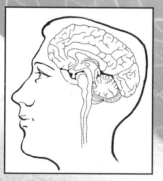

The brain stem controls the basic life functions such as respiration, circulation, and digestion. The brain stem consists of various brain structures. The brain stem is associated with the 6TH Chakra.

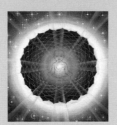

Complete Unity of Body, Emotions, and Soul

A thousand-leaf, lavender lotus flower symbolizes the seventh Chakra. This Chakra symbolizes perfect harmony and complete integration of body, emotion, mind, and spirit.

The seventh Chakra creates truth and happiness in their purest essence. Here, a sense of the individual self disappears. Awareness is from a place of truth, and everything is in holistic unity, without the illusion of separation. This allows you to fully experience the harmonious order of the cosmos.

An individual with an inactive seventh Chakra will not be able to experience spiritual existence, nor understand the realm of the soul and the universe. Inability to acknowledge the spiritual aspect of life means ignorance of the essential purpose of life.

It is not possible to explain the awakening of the seventh Chakra with words. Nor is it possible to analyze it in logical or scientific terms. The seventh Chakra is a place of infinity, allowing the state of Oneness, where suffering caused by illusory pleasure, pain, fame, and wealth is non-existent. To find your own divinity, to reach a state of salvation, and to reach Nirvana all refer to a full awakening of the seventh Chakra.

Chakra Activation with the
Power Brain Energizer

Through regular vibratory stimulation, the Power Brain Energizer can effectively awaken and activate the individual Chakras. The frequency of the Power Brain Energizer vibration lowers the brain waves to facilitate the enhancement of energy. The Power Brain Energizer can help you awaken each Chakra so that you can easily retain and recall the specific sensations associated with each Chakra.

We begin by stimulating the Jang-shim Chakra points on the hands, before moving on to the seven internal Chakras. Then, we move from the first to the seventh Chakra in reverse order.

1 Sit comfortably in half lotus position, with your shoulders relaxed. Turn the Power Brain Energizers on, and place them in your hands. Raise your hands two inches above your knees.

2 Focus on the vibration in your hands and then slowly move your hands in a circular motion. Expand the feeling of vibration from your hands to your arms, shoulders, chest, abdomen, neck, and Dahn-jon.

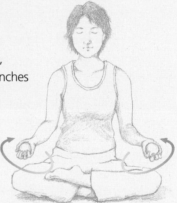

3 Now, turn the Power Brain Energizer on your left hand off while leaving the right one on. Place the Power Brain Energizer on your Baek-hwe and focus on the vibration. Turn the Power Brain Energizer off and retain the memory of the vibration, while visualizing the vibration coursing through your brain.

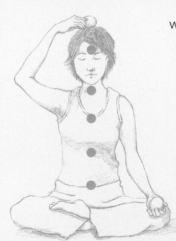

4 Now, turn the Power Brain Energizer on again and place it against your In-dang point. Focus on the vibration entering the In-dang, as it moves deep inside your brain. Turn the Power Brain Energizer off and feel the lingering vibration...

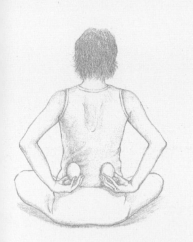

5 Turn the Power Brain Energizer on and place it against your neck, feeling the vibration spread out into your brain and shoulders. Massage the whole area in order to increase the stimulation. Turn the Power Brain Energizer off and retain the feeling of the vibration for as long as possible.

6 Relax your shoulders and place the Power Brain Energizer against your sternum. Breathe in as you feel the vibration cover your whole chest, and then breathe out forcefully. Massage the whole area of the fourth Chakra with the Power Brain Energizer. Feel the vibration travel downward to your elbows and then to your hands. Turn the Power Brain Energizer off and recall the sensation.

7 Turn the Power Brain Energizer on and place it against the Joong-wahn point in your upper abdomen, two inches above your navel. Feel the vibration reach into your stomach and internal organs, facilitating circulation. Turn the Power Brain Energizer off and recall the sensation.

8 Turn the Power Brain Energizer on and place it against your lower Dahn-jon. Focus on the vibration that courses through the whole lower abdomen. Feel the intestines stir as your abdomen fills with deep warmth. Turn the Power Brain Energizer off and recall the sensation. Turn the Power Brain Energizer on again and place it on your back, near your kidneys... then place it over the approximate locations of other internal organs. Feel the flow of energy in your stomach, liver, and kidneys...

9 Now, turn the Power Brain Energizer on and place it against your Hwe-um, using your body weight to secure it in place. Feel the vibration spread out from your Hwe-um to the rest of your pelvis, traveling up along your spine, all the way to the seventh Chakra. Focus on the feeling of the vibration moving throughout your body.

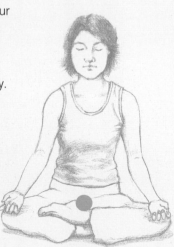

10 Breathe in... and breathe out, and sit in half lotus position. Turn the Power Brain Energizers on and place them on your hands. Focus on the feeling of the vibration as it travels through your arms to the fourth Chakra, then down to the first Chakra, and then to the Yong-chun points at the bottoms of your feet. Visualize your energy body riding along the wave of vibration. Feel the strengthening of the energy body.

3. Activating the Chakras (Vibration)

Vibration is the easiest and most effective way of awakening and activating the Chakras. It is more efficient to activate the whole Chakra system at once through vibration training, rather than activating each Chakra one by one. A prerequisite to activating the Chakras is the unimpeded and free flow of energy throughout the body. Vibration training is the most effective way of achieving an uninterrupted energy flow. Self-vibration training is an excellent way to activate the first through fourth Chakras. Once the four lower Chakras are active, the remaining Chakras become active just from the power of the lower four.

When doing vibration training, we each develop a certain resonant frequency to our vibration. This frequency is the natural rhythm of our body and coincides with the natural rhythm of life of the universe. It is at that moment that we begin to feel the sensation of Yullyo come alive within us. Once a palpable sensation of Yullyo courses through us, our natural healing powers are stronger because Yullyo restores harmony.

A sick cell has a different resonant frequency than a healthy cell.

In fact, the reason for illness is that cells, or an organ, have lost their natural frequency. Through vibration training, we can recover the lost, natural frequency, and thereby restore health to afflicted areas of the body.

Self-vibration training is like Dahn-mu in practice. Dahn-mu occurs spontaneously as you trace the subtle sensation of energy in your hands. Likewise, Self-vibration training occurs spontaneously when you stop the flow of conscious thought and apply vibratory stimulation to your body. It is essential that you eliminate thinking during Self-vibration training, since self-vibration occurs in the absence of mental activity. During Dahn-mu, people tend to experience an absence of thoughts, leading to inner peace and joy that arises when following paths of energy. During Self-vibration training, you must let yourself go and embrace the natural vibration of life that emanates from deep inside the brain stem.

The primary reason for difficulty with Self-vibration training is the inability to let go of inhibition or self-consciousness of the left-brain. This separates you from the flow of the universal life force. Only when you let go of your conscious thoughts can you communicate with that universal life force and experience the Yullyo within. Therefore, Healing Chakra training begins with letting go of your thoughts.

However, when you first begin Self-vibration training, some form of conscious effort is necessary to get going. First, stimulate the Yong-chun points in the center of the bottom of your feet in order to generate a certain vibration, which will then radiate out to the Chakras above. When you feel your body begin to generate a rhythm, let go and immerse yourself in that rhythm with joy and abandon.

In the beginning, play bright, rhythmic music to start the self-vibration process. Once you have developed a naturally occurring rhythm, concentrate only on the movements of your body. Close your eyes and listen to the music. Let the rhythm of the music merge with your own rhythm until you feel your body move with, and then become, the rhythm itself. This is the most comfortable and natural state we can experience.

Beginning Self-Vibration Chakra Training

Stand with your feet shoulder width apart,
With your arms loose and relaxed along your sides.
Let a light smile float upon your face.
With a slight flex of the knees,
Spring up and down lightly on your toes.

Concentrate on your Yong-chun points,
Located on the bottoms of your feet...
Feel the energy of the earth
Flow upward through your legs, though your knees...
Yong-chun... Yong-chun... Yong-chun...
Shift your consciousness slowly from
the Yong-chun to your ankles.
Ankles... Ankles... Ankles...
From your ankles to your knees...

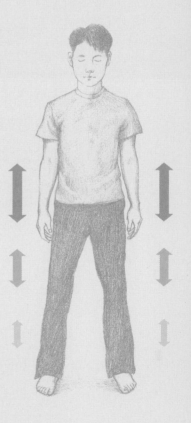

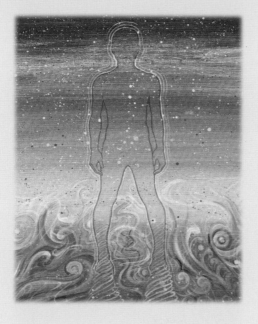

Continue moving your body up and down
Focusing on the music and rhythm...
Allow the natural rhythm to spread to your knees
Moving up and down.
You feel your muscles working.
Knees... Knees... Knees...
Now focus on your hips,
Expanding the sensation throughout your legs,
Until the lower body vibrates
With your own unique rhythm of life...

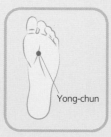

Yong-chun

Self-Vibration Chakra Training

Let the vibration touch the first Chakra,
Located in the Hwe-um...
Hwe-um... Hwe-um... Hwe-um
Touch your tongue lightly to the roof of your mouth.
Feel the vibration in your Hwe-um.
The vibration gradually expands upwards into the lower Dahn-jon.
Concentrate on the second Chakra, the lower Dahn-jon.
Dahn-jon... Dahn-jon... Dahn-jon...
Feel the vibration in your uterus, bladder,
Awaken the sensation of the second Chakra.
Move your waist to the front, back, and sides,
Expanding the vibration...

Feel the energy travel
Up and down your Hwe-um and lower Dahn-jon,

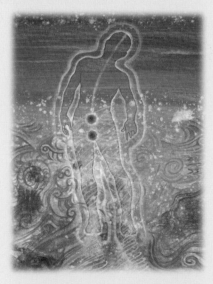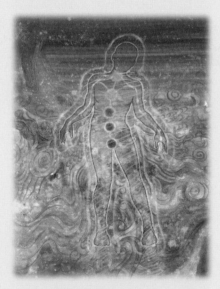

Moving your whole body up and down.
Feel your intestines twist and uncurl,
As your waist moves around and around.
As the second Chakra becomes warm,
You can feel a stream of cold energy
Flowing out through your Hwe-um...
The vibration that began in your tailbone
Now travels upward to each vertebra of the spine,
Stimulating and caressing each one,
All the way to your neck...
The energy from your head
Flows down to the Hwe-um and Dahn-jon,
Leaving your head cool and your Dahn-jon warm...

Now concentrate on the third Chakra,
Just above the navel at the point of the Joong-wahn.
The energy lying stagnant in the stomach
Begins to unfurl and move.
Stomach... liver... kidneys...
Energy is connecting the organs and creating warmth.
Now concentrate on the fourth Chakra, on your Dahn-joong.
Let the vibration take hold of your arms and shoulders.
The energy lying stagnant in the chest
Flows outward through your palms and fingertips...

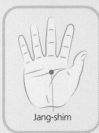

Jang-shim

Now concentrate on the fifth Chakra, in your throat.
Your head may move from side to side,
Rotating to the left and right...
Let the stagnant energy flow outward
Through the Jang-shim points in your palms...

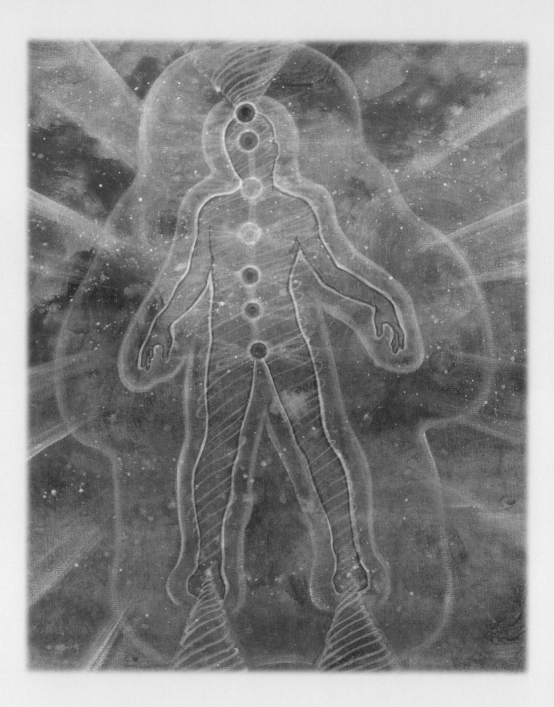

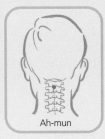

Ah-mun

(Concentrate for two or three minutes on the sensation of each Chakra:
Dahn-jon - Joong-wahn - Dahn-joong - Throat)
Let the vibration ring from the Ah-mun point to the top of your head.
Feel your lips, tongue and face...
Feel every cell, every organ, every blood vessel vibrate...
Feel your whole body tremble with the joy of energy
Connecting your body's Chakras
From your tailbone to the top of your head...
Immerse yourself wholly in the currents of energy,
And let the energy flow through any blockages.
You may feel strong vibration around the blocked areas.
Your spine unwinds with the flow and your back straightens.
Your head and neck move and rotate freely,
As your hands tap your chest...
Your body moves and shakes
You might try beating your chest
To the joyful rhythm of life's natural resonance
Being expressed through your body...
(15 to 20 minutes is the approximate amount
of time for this Self-vibration training)

Concluding Self-Vibration Chakra Training

Now gradually stop the vibration.
Bring your hands with palms up to your Dahn-jon.
Leave your left hand near your Dahn-jon.
Slowly bring your right hand
Up to the seventh Chakra while you breathe in.

Turn your right hand over so that it faces the ground.
As you breathe out,
Bring it down all the way to your lower Dahn-jon,
Sweeping down the length of your torso...
Repeat this motion three times.

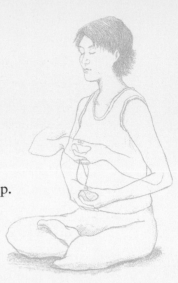

Now sit in half lotus position with your palms facing up.
Breathe in as you bring your hands to chest level.
Breathe out as you lower your hands to
Your Dahn-jon once more.
Repeat this until you feel your body enter
A state of comfortable relaxation.
Then lower your hands onto your knees.
Conclude the training by
Internally observing each individual Chakra.

Chakra Vibration and 'Voicing'

'Voicing' is using sound vibration to awaken the Chakras. Self-vibration is most effective in awakening and activating the lower four Chakras, while Voicing is more effective in stimulating the upper three Chakras.

Voicing brings energy out from deep within to give it sound, thereby stimulating the body's internal organs and cells with a subtle vibration. Like Self-vibration, Voicing relaxes the muscles and facilitates the flow of Ki energy through the body. The "Om" sound is especially effective in directly stimulating the brain to maintain balance and harmony among all the internal organs. By lowering the active brain waves, Voicing has the effect of dissolving emotional fluctuations, including those from fear and grief. The sound "Om" has traditionally been the sound of Oneness, symbolizing the essential unity of all. Voicing, when practiced deeply, can become a way to experience divinity.

Sit or stand in a comfortable position and relax.
Place your hands in front of your heart in prayer position.
Lightly touch your tongue to the roof of your mouth.
Close your eyes and give voice to the sound, "Om~."
Elongate the voicing of the "Om~" sound
As if you are drawing energy up from the first Chakra.
Let the vibration from the first Chakra
Continue through each Chakra,
Arriving at the seventh...
Continue voicing the "Om~" sound,
And feel the subtle vibration
In the cells and organs of your body.
You might even feel your brain stir...
The vibration becomes stronger,
Moving your body to the rhythm
Of your own voice...

Let yourself move to the naturally
Occurring rhythm,
And continue voicing the "Om~" sound...
Imagine the vibration from your body
Radiating out, expanding...
Imagine each cell pulsating
Rhythmically to your voice.

The sound of "Om~" is ringing throughout the cosmos,
As you ride the waves,
Expanding the horizon of your awareness...

Imagine the whole universe filled with vibration of the sound
As you become One with cosmic awareness.
Shaking joyfully with the vibration of your voice,
Each Chakra blossoms spontaneously.
Each Chakra, a lotus flower of a different form...
Observe your body silently, feel the energy body...
Healthy, happy, and peaceful...
Feel your heart... with joy and peace radiating outward...

Feel the warm flow from your Dahn-jon.
From where does such joy and peace come?
This warmth and comfort you feel is the sensation of life.
You are meeting life within.
This life that exists within you
Is the real you,
Existing before the body
Alive before your name...
Life existing of itself, by itself, and in itself...
Within it, you experience infinite peace.
Now, lower your hands to your knees.
Slowly let your consciousness float to the surface...

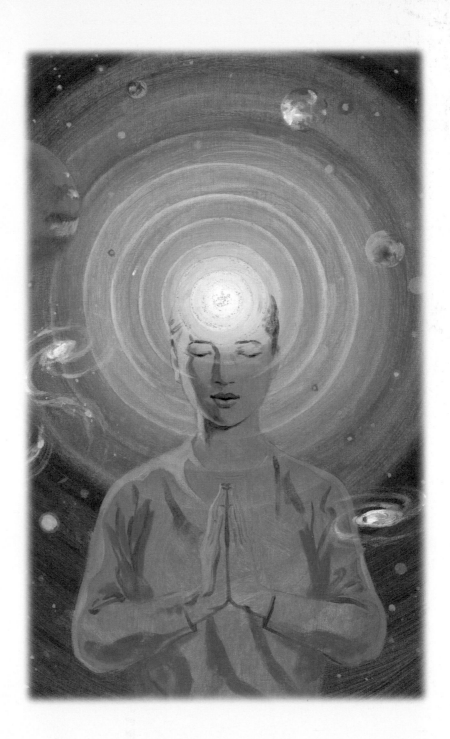

4. Strengthening the Chakras

The aura is an energy field around our body. It envelops the body fully, and is generated by the Chakras. Our aura accurately reflects the state of our body and mind. A weak and hazy aura reflects a malfunctioning Chakra system. In a person with a healthy, fully functioning Chakra system, the aura is bright and strong.

Surrounding energy affects Chakras and aura systems. When standing next to a person who has a healthy Chakra system, your own Chakras become stronger. On the other hand, standing next to a depressed person may elicit a feeling of depression in you. Very sensitive people can feel a specific part of their body ache when standing next to a person who has pain in the corresponding place.

It is impossible to avoid the influence of surrounding energies in the world. Although you may start out with a healthy Chakra system, it can lose harmony due to exposure to unbalanced energy. However, you need not become a hermit in order to maintain a healthy Chakra system. To protect the auric field, it is possible to develop a protective energy capsule around your body. This allows you to maintain a close relationship with people while at the same time, purifying and protecting your own energy system.

An energy capsule is different from the naturally occurring aura, in that it occurs through conscious awareness and consists of the fundamental vibration of the universe. A small, circular hole exists in the energy capsule on top of the Baek-hwe point that connects you to a supply of fresh, positive energy from the universe. Directly in front of this column of energy, there is a smaller hole of about 1/3 inch that pumps negative and stagnant energy out of the body. With this capsule, it is possible to protect and purify yourself while inter-acting with the world. Capsule training is especially effective when practiced early in the morning and late at night just before you go to sleep. Practicing Capsule training before you fall asleep helps you to rest more deeply, and thus to economize on sleeping time. When feeling tired and fatigued during the day, you can recharge yourself by picturing the capsule and consciously receiving energy.

When our Chakra system is active and fully functioning, and our spiritual awareness approaches cosmic awareness, our energy body takes on the color of brightly radiating gold. A golden energy body has a powerful loving and healing force, acting to purify neg-ativity. When our awareness becomes one with cosmic awareness, our energy body glows with a whitish silver color of indescribable brightness.

Making an Energy Glove

Raise your hands and gently shake them.
Feel the air passing through your fingers,
Over and under your hands...

Continue shaking your hands until you feel
A tangible sensation of energy envelop them.

Now, stop shaking your hands.
Focus on the energy field,
As it forms along the tips of your fingers...
Keep concentrating and you will feel
Electricity, or heat... on both hands.
Feel the energy flow inward through your fingertips...
Focus on the energy flow,
From your hands to your wrists and elbows...
All the way up to your shoulders...

Breathe in as you raise both hands,
Palms facing up, to shoulder level...
Then lower them again as you exhale.
Link the motion of your hands
To the rhythm of your breathing...
Your hands will move up and down
Without conscious thinking on your part...
Control your breath with your mind,
Control your energy with your mind.
Your breath will deepen and become slower.
Feel the breath from your chest move
To your Dahn-jon... then down to your feet,
Spreading outward in all directions,
Until it reaches every cell in your body,
Each cell breathing in and out...
This is how your mind moves energy.
It is how energy moves the body.

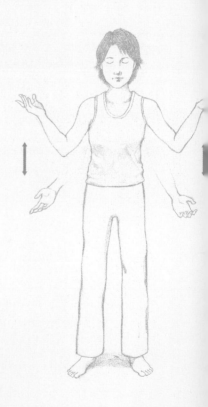

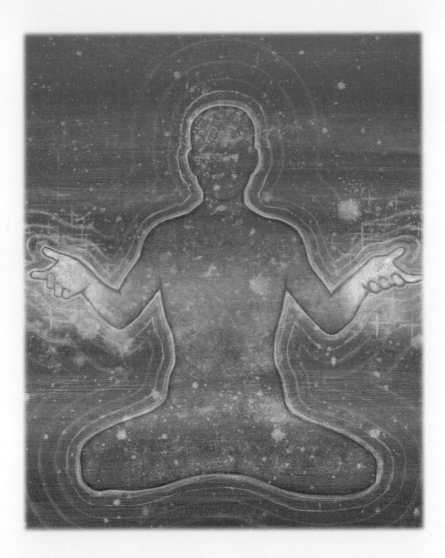

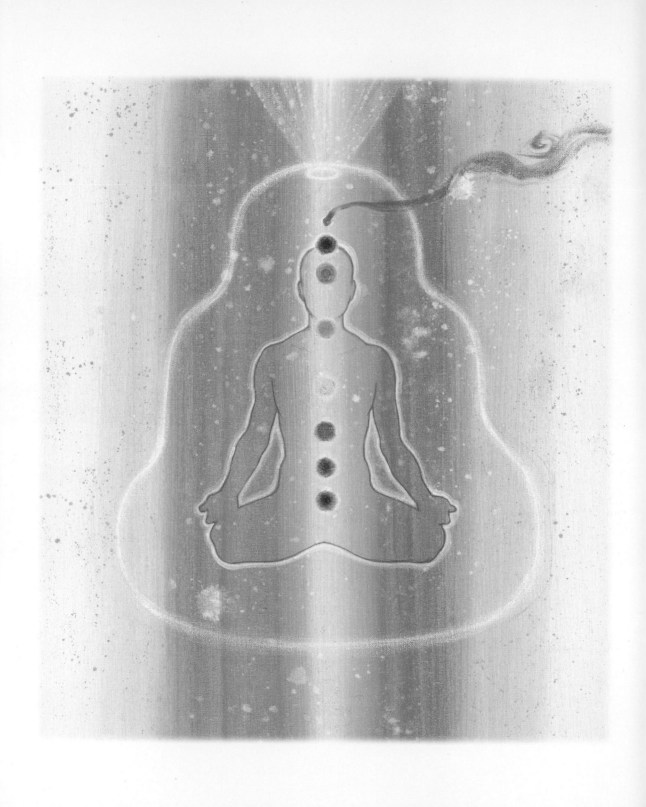

Generating a Capsule of Energy

Keeping the feeling of energy that surrounds your hands alive,
Bring your hands close to your face...
When your hands are about four inches from your face,
Wash your face with Ki energy,
Without touching it, but with the living sensation
Of warm energy enveloping your face...

Sweep from your face to the back of your head
Elongating the energy sheath...
Now sweep and cover both arms with this energy sheath.
Then sweep from your chest to your waist, to your legs...
You are putting on a veil of energy.

Now imagine a thick, pulsating energy capsule,
About eight inches from your skin,
Surround your whole body.

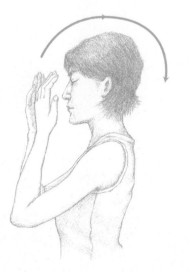
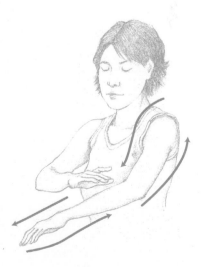

Imagine a small hole on top of your Baek-hwe
Into which pure silver-white energy flows.
In this way, you can fill yourself with energy whenever you wish.
Imagine a smaller hole in front of the Baek-hwe
From which stagnant energy escapes.

Breathe and feel the capsule, cleansing and purifying.
Within the capsule, your body and mind
Are restored to original purity and health...

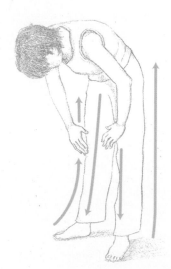

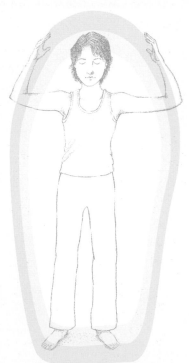

Strengthening the Energy Capsule through Chakra Training

Stand with your legs shoulder width apart
With your knees bent at about 15 degrees.
Raise your hands to chest level,
As if holding a large barrel in your arms...
Feel the energy of the earth travel up to your knees.
Energy enters the Yong-chun on the bottom of your feet,
Passing through the Hwe-um in the first Chakra,
And gathering in the second Chakra.

Now, through the seventh Chakra,
You feel a connection to the energy of heaven.
The energies of heaven and earth meet in your Dahn-jon.
To strengthen the sensation of energy,
Imagine a heavy boulder on top of your head.
Imagine the ground rising to lift up your feet.
Feeling the pressure of heaven and earth
Link the energies from your toes to your head.

Your body stands upright with the strength of heaven and earth,
Becoming a passageway for the energy.
Focus on your spine... and feel a solid pillar of energy
That connects your tailbone to your Baek-hwe.
As you breathe in and out, feel the pillar becoming thicker.
Now, inhale and hold your breath for five seconds,
Feeling the pillar of energy... growing thicker still...
Now breathe out, and feel the energy pillar growing thinner...
Breathe in again, and tighten your sphincter muscle.

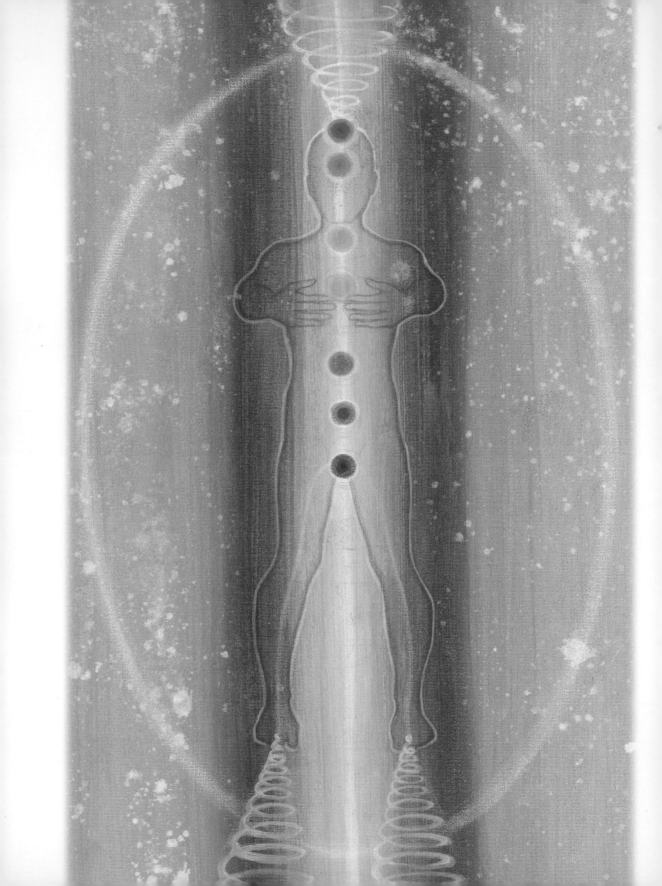

Feel the energy rise from your tailbone to your Baek-hwe
As you hold your breath.
Now breathe out once again,
Feeling the Chakras along your spine.
Breathe in and out...
Until you feel the Chakras coming alive.
Holding your breath for ten seconds
Will strengthen the sensation.

Now, place both hands over the second Chakra,
About four inches from your skin...
Place a field of warm energy,
Soothing and massaging, over your Dahn-jon...
Let the energy of the earth flow upward
Through your Yong-chun, to your knees,
And into your Hwe-um...
Twisting and turning like a tornado
And gathering in your Dahn-jon.

Pure energy of the heavens flows in through
Your Baek-hwe,
Passing through the In-dang,
Joong-wahn, and Dahn-jon...
The energy from the earth below
And the energy from the heavens above
Meet in your Dahn-jon in a swirling
Of Yin and Yang...
Now, silently feel the warmth of these energies...
And expand the swirling sensation of energy
To envelop all of you,

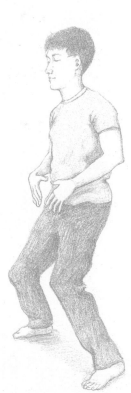

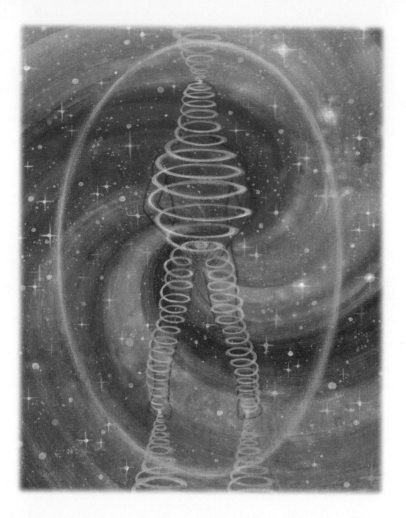

Until you palpably feel its presence.

As you breathe in and out...

The energy capsule becomes stronger and brighter.

5. Healing the Chakras

I f only one of the seven Chakras develops and becomes active, the whole system becomes unbalanced. A person repeatedly engaged in mental activity while working has a well-developed system of upper Chakras. Without working to maintain balance, the lower Chakras will weaken, increasing susceptibility to depression or other types of mental instability. The lower body will also weaken physically.

Two ways of restoring harmonious balance to the body are through self-healing and healing with a partner. Both methods require the ability to feel the Chakras and the energy body. However, it is even possible for beginners to engage in these healing practices. It is important for a beginner to trust his or her own sensitivity. Take some time to observe your partner, observing his or her energy. Pay attention to the color, temperature, brightness and clarity of the Chakras. Begin to sense the stream of information coming from the other person.

In the lower three Chakras, there is a feeling of warmth from the color red. From the fifth to the seventh Chakras, there is a feeling of cool blueness. On the fourth Chakra, you can feel a balance of red and blue, in both color and warmth. A problem with the lower Chakras transmits as a cold sensation that is white or bluish-black. A problem in the upper Chakras presents itself as a hot sensation of dark, angry red. While this may seem difficult at first, with practice and confidence, you will be able to read the Chakras accurately.

As you place a sheath of energy on another person, you can sense the state of his or her energy body. Problems with the energy body are conveyed by dark or cold sensations, or a sense of hesitation in the formation of the energy capsule. When you feel coldness over a particular part, remove it, and infuse the exact location with warmth. When you find an area of the energy sheath that is thin, infuse that area with concentrated energy. When you feel stagnant or negative energy, draw the energy out and replace it with fresh energy.

There are two methods of communicating energy to others. One technique entails placing your hand about two inches from the receiver, and moving it back and forth with a rhythmic, spring-like motion. You can also transmit energy by rotating your hand in a clockwise direction, again, keeping your hands two inches from the receiver. The giver of energy should have his or her eyes open while the receiver has his or her eyes closed. Both partners should be in a state of patient receptivity. Purity of intention is necessary for healing. Give energy with love and sincerity. Receive energy with gratitude and trust.

Self-Healing

Shower of Light

Close your eyes and stand or sit comfortably,
With your neck and back straight.
Visualize a bright, golden sun
Suspended just above your head...
Imagine its golden rays showering down on
The crown of your head.
The lotus flower of the seventh Chakra
Slowly opens its petals,
Tasting the golden delight of the sun.
You feel a tingling sensation
On top of your Baek-hwe,
Bathed by a shower of golden light.
Its warmth moves through your body
And reaches your first Chakra.
A clean line of golden energy
Forms a pillar of light connecting
your seven Chakras.

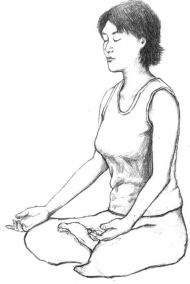

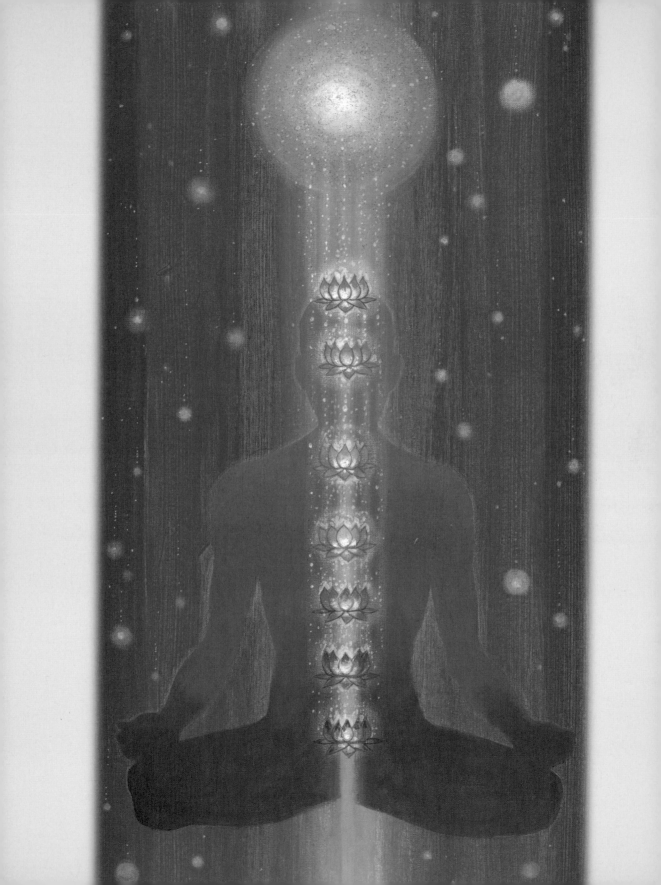

Now, imagine the sun
Shining in front of your face...
Dazzling, yet soft...
Warm and comforting...
Feel the light enter your In-dang,
Lighting up your eyes...
Now feel the energy touch upon your fifth Chakra,
Imparting a feeling of warmth to your neck.
Move down the Chakra ladder...
Fourth, third, second, and first...
Allowing each one to feel the golden light of the sun...
Immerse yourself in the field of golden rays
As they cleanse and purify every cell,
Filling you with the pure energy of the universe.

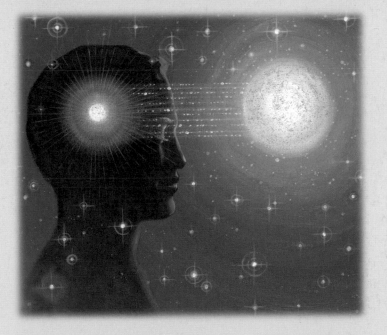

Transmitting Energy with Your Hands

Now bring your hands to your chest, hands two inches apart...
Focus on your hands, feeling the field of energy coming alive.
Rub your hands together without touching...
Feel the energy field becoming stronger.
Place your right hand about four inches From the top of your head.
Concentrate on the energy emanating from the seventh Chakra.
Feel a vortex of golden energy radiating from your hands,
And spiraling down towards the Baek-hwe,
Imparting a feeling of warmth and presence.

Now bring your hand in front of your In-dang
And transmit energy to your sixth Chakra.
Feel the gentle tendrils of the energy field
Reaching out and enveloping.
Now, bring your hands to the sides of your head
Near your temples and transmit energy...
Allow the energy to seep deeply into your brain stem...

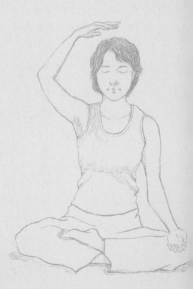

Lower your hands to your neck
Feeling the energy of the fifth Chakra...
If you are having problems with your thyroid glands,
Send blue-colored energy through your hands.
Continue sending the energy until your neck
Is ringed by a collar of blue energy.
Come down to the fourth Chakra
And transmit energy to your chest.
If you are having problems with your heart or lungs,
Or feel a blockage along the front meridian,

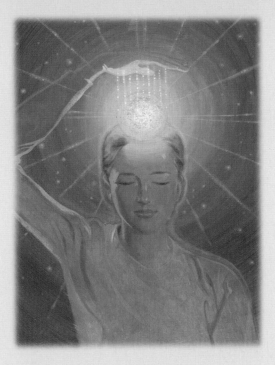

Then imagine golden energy
Reaching out to embrace your heart and lungs.

A problem with the first, second, or third Chakra
Will give the appearance of a white or blackish red color.
Sense the color, light, and temperature of each Chakra.
If you feel cold, dark strands, pluck them out one by one.
If you sense some weakness,
Then transmit additional energy.
After a while, you will experience a feeling
Of soft energy flowing to your hands.
If you feel an energy blockage in an area,
Transmit energy as you rotate your hand clockwise,
Until you break through the barrier,
Activating and freeing trapped energy.

Partner-Healing

Sensing the Energy Field of a Partner

Stand facing your partner
Left palms facing skyward,
Right palms facing the ground.
Bring your hands about two inches away
From your partner's palms.
Close your eyes and feel the energy field
Of one another...
Hands moving closer together...
Then further apart...
Strengthening the bond of mutual energy.

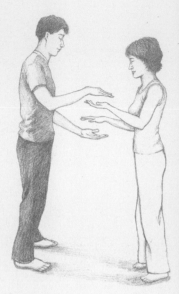

Now, one partner lowers her arms
And stands in a relaxed position.
With both hands about two inches
From your partner's body,
Feel the energy field of different areas of the body,
Including the shoulders, arms, chest, and legs...
Then, begin from the bottom and come back up again,
Feeling the energy field of your partner's back.
Repeat this three times,
Until you have a clear sense of the energy field
That surrounds your partner.
Focus on the subtle vibration of energy
That you can sense with your fingertips.
Then, discuss the condition of the energy field
With your partner.

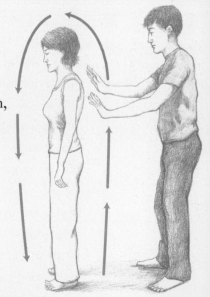

Putting an Energy Capsule on a Partner

Now let's place an energy capsule around your partner
To purify and heal the areas
Of disharmony and imbalance.
First, rub your hands together to gather energy.
Standing about ten inches from your partner,
Surround your partner with a capsule of energy.
Using the energy of your hands, begin with the face.
Move down the front and up the back of your partner as before.
This time, instead of just feeling the energy,
Place a sheath of energy over your partner.
Wrap a capsule of healing energy around your partner...
From top to bottom...

Concentrate on your partner's individual Chakras
Throughout this process.
You may feel a cool draft or a stream of warmth.
Coolness signifies lack of circulation,
And may create a prickling sensation in your hands.
In some areas, you may feel a thick stream
Or lump of energy.
In other areas, energy may be subtle
And barely perceptible.
Certain areas may resist the capsule,
And create a sensation of dissolving the energy.
Focus your energy on these areas,
And pass your hands over them repeatedly.
Trust your energy sensitivity, instinct
And insight to move your hands,

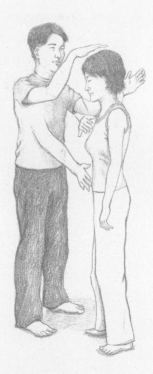

Stopping the flow of thoughts, intellect, and judgment.
Once you completely trust in your ability to sense energy,
Your hands will move of their own accord.
They will find weak and painful spots,
Reinforcing areas in need of energy.
Let your hands be guided by the sensation of energy,
Further assisted by the guidance of your soul,
Purifying and supplying energy...

Sweeping downward from the Baek-hwe,
Focus on the sensation of the seventh, sixth, and fifth Chakras.
If you sense darkness or coolness in the fifth Chakra,
There may be a problem with the thyroid glands.
Draw the stream of coolness out of the neck
As if you were pulling on a thread.
Then replenish it with fresh energy.
When you perceive a sense of balance in the area,
Move down to the next Chakra.
Feel the state of the fourth Chakra with your hands.
If you sense coolness, darkness, or prickling,
Draw the negative energies out with your hands.

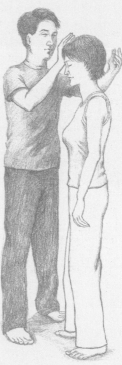

When working on the third Chakra or below,
Bend your knees so that you are comfortable.
Sense the temperature of the first and second Chakras.
If you feel a cool draft,
Counter it with a blast of warm energy from your hands,
Until you feel the area covered with warmth.

Repeat the motions of this chakra healing three times.
You will feel the energy field become stronger and purer
Each time you pass over your partner's body.
Afterward, briskly sweep down the whole body.
With your partner,
Discuss what each of you felt during the process.
Through this, your sensitivity to Ki energy will increase,
And your healing powers will be enhanced.

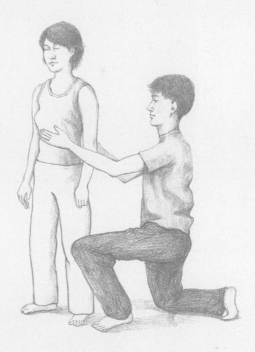

Using the **Power Brain Energizer**
for Partner-Healing

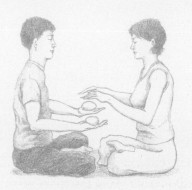

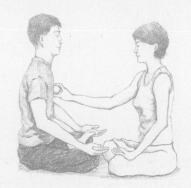

1 Sit facing your partner. Turn the Power Brain Energizers on and place them in your partner's hands. Hold your hands, palms down, one inch above your partner's hands.

2 Now, put one Power Brain Energizer aside and place the other against your partner's fourth Chakra, or Dahn-joong, located near the sternum. Have your partner close his or her eyes. Slowly and gently massage the Dahn-joong with the Power Brain Energizer.

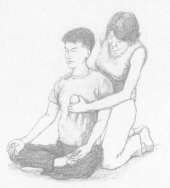

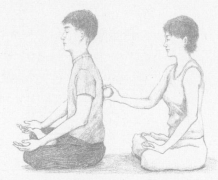

3 Let your hand guide you to places in your partner's body against which to place the Power Brain Energizer, with the exception of the Baek-hwe. Stimulate the chosen areas for five seconds each.

4 Place the Power Brain Energizer on your partner's spine, remaining for about one minute in each section. Feel for areas that are weak, stiff, or tense, and focus your treatment in those areas.

106

6. Chakra Meditation

Chakra meditation is designed to bring you back to zero, to neutrality, to a place of balance. The ultimate purpose of Healing Chakra training is to free your soul. Most people live out their lives without recognizing the existence of the soul within. Emotions, thoughts, preconceptions... these things are not your soul. Yet, many people mistake these things for their soul. Throughout our lives, we are bombarded with an endless stream of information that prevents our souls from being free. Our dislikes, as well as our desires, cage our souls.

Freedom of your soul begins the moment you empty the vessel of your soul. The weight of the soul is zero, to begin with. A soul is free only when it stands in the place of zero. Only when you return to zero are you able to freely choose again. When you feel a heaviness of your soul, you are still holding on to something.

Just for this moment, let go of all thoughts, preconceptions, and emotions. Let your body move according to the flow of energy. Then you will hear the voice of your soul.

Listening to the Message of the Soul

Sit in half lotus position and close your eyes.
Imagine a single lotus flower
As it takes root in your body and blossoms forth.
The stalk of the lotus rises along your spine,
Its roots embedded in the Hwe-um.
The bud of the lotus flower lies softly
On top of the seventh Chakra...
As you breathe in, let your consciousness
Travel from the root of the lotus flower
To the bud of the lotus flower...
As you breathe out, let your consciousness
Travel downward... to the Hwe-um.
Let the flower return to a bud while breathing in,

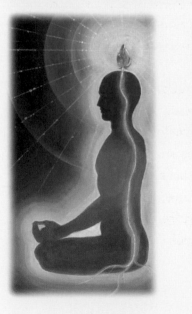
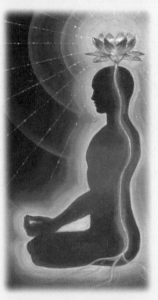

And blossom forth again as you breathe out...

As your breathing deepens, the flower opens wide,
Its roots extending in all directions...
As the flower blossoms, your soul blooms beautifully,
Communicating freely with cosmic energy,
Bringing the message of the cosmos
Through the beauty of the lotus flower...

Now, with both hands, envelop the sixth Chakra.
A golden light is seeping
Through your sixth Chakra, Heaven's Palace...
Energy emanating from your hands
Is going into the cells deep inside your brain.
It softly soothes the brain stem,
Awakening the pure soul sleeping therein.
Meet the light of life
That existed before your name
In the palace of the sixth Chakra...

"I am eternal, without beginning or end."
"I am light, sound, and vibration existing by itself."
"Light, sound, and vibration are my reality."
"Until now, my soul was imprisoned by a name."
"Until now, my soul was caged by a body."
"Now I am free of my body... and my name..."

From the Baek-hwe, In-dang, and the temples...
From the four points of your head,
You are drawing out the energy

Of darkness and stagnation.
Bars that imprison the soul,
Fear, doubt, hatred, attachment...
Draw out all of these energies.
Brighten your sixth Chakra
With a silvery-white light,
Translucent and beautiful...

Now imagine the cosmic energy
Connecting the sixth and seventh Chakras,
As the brightly shining Big Dipper
Descends into your Baek-hwe and In-dang.
Let your soul assume the shape of a bird
And fly from the lotus flower of the seventh Chakra...
The soul, pure and white
Freed from the bars of preconceptions and attachment,
Flies away into the blue sky...
Your soul exists with true freedom
In the infinite space of the cosmos...
Breathe in and out three times...
And raise your consciousness slowly to the surface.

Pure Consciousness Meditation

This training is to bring separated divinity into the original Oneness. Through the process of meditation, you will bring body and mind, logic and emotion, False-Self and True-Self, and all other forms of duality together. As you meditate in this position, your breath will deepen naturally and your body will be replenished with energy.

Touch your fingertips together. Since all meridians of the body are connected through the fingertips, this brings all energies of the organs and Chakras together. The place of emptiness is the place where duality no longer exists. This is the place of pure consciousness where cleansing and purification occur. This meditation will return you to yourself, beyond all space and time. This meditation will allow you to meet with the essence of life before it had a name. You may practice this meditation in any comfortable position, sitting or standing.

Concentrate on your Dahn-jon
With your back straight and shoulders relaxed.
Bring your fingertips together
In front of your chest
And form them into a ball.
Through the fingertips,
All organs are connected
And all Chakras are bonded.
Current flows through your fingertips
And warmth greets each finger.
Your mind is truly at rest
As golden light fills your hands...
Imagine another you hidden within the light.

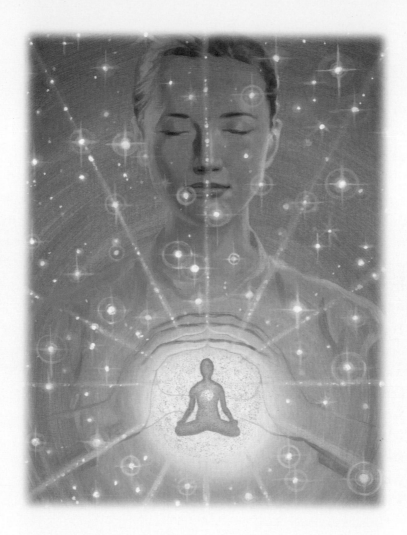

You are there,
Inside the golden aura of the cosmos...

Observe yourself floating in space,
Pure and unadulterated as at birth,
Neither man nor woman...
Without name or title...
Pure life... is what you observe.
You are infinitely peaceful,
Within a space inviolable to all,
A space of pure consciousness...

From this place of pure consciousness,
Body and mind find harmony
And all memories of suffering dissolve,
Returning you to the place of zero.
Body and mind become pure and clean
In this place of emptiness...
You return to the place of original being,
Where true shape is the purity of the soul
That exists within you always.
Whenever you wish, you may return here
To purify your body and mind...

Change Your Energy

Change Your Brain

Change Your Life

Part IV
Everyday Healing Chakra

In the course of our lives

We encounter several opportunities

To hear the voice of our soul...

Wake up when you hear the sound

And speak with your soul...

Complete your journey.

1. Chakra Brain Respiration

Every color has its own unique frequency and energy. Psychological and physical responses to different colors are already the subject of much study, with some colors being used for healing purposes. The colors of the Chakras incorporate the spectrum of the rainbow, making it impossible to define a specific, definite color for one Chakra. The actual colors sensed during Healing Chakra training will vary among individuals. This is why books or meditation groups differ in their choice of colors of the Chakras.

Passion, creation, life, love, peace, wisdom, and completion... these energies are essential to living. By meditating on these words and concepts everyday, you can create happiness and joy. You can be reborn everyday with renewed body and mind. It is the energy of your mind and consciousness that heals you. For your mind and consciousness are the mind and consciousness of the cosmos. "My Energy is Cosmic Energy; My Mind is Cosmic Mind." This is what I shouted at the moment of enlightenment. This is truth as I have experienced it.

If you practice the type of meditation described here, you will not only be able to heal yourself, but also your neighbors, society, and the world. You will become a bright light in your community. When you are at a crossroads, when you feel down or lacking in energy, when you feel confused and chaotic... when you need the power of the cosmos... just reach out with your hand, and in return, you will receive health of body and mind.

Chakra Brain Respiration is a training method designed to awaken the infinite potential of the brain by activating the Chakras through color. We will use the unique vibration of each color to stimulate each individual Chakra, which in turn stimulates the brain. When engaging in Chakra Brain Respiration, you can choose a color according to your condition. You can choose a different color for each day of the week, since there are seven to choose from. You will then feel your life filled with energy. Use the Healing Chakra booklet that accompanies this book to help you visualize the colors for a more effective training session.

1. Sit in a comfortable position and relax your body. Set up the individual Healing Chakra picture about 20 inches from your eyes. Choose the color you want for the day. Observe the picture calmly and silently, feeling the sensation of the color... cold, hot, warm... comfortable... disturbing... soothing...

2. Now, close your eyes and imagine the picture you've just seen. Let the picture become larger and brighter in your mind's eye, infusing your whole being with its light. Let the light cascade over you... allowing the light to be absorbed by your body, exploding in intensity as it hits the corresponding Chakra. If you want passion in your life, repeat the words, "Passion... passion..." as you visualize the color red. Feel the sensation of the

particular frequency of vibration that corresponds to the color you have chosen.

3. Now, breathe the color in... and breathe out. Accept the color as you breathe it in, then expel all the negative energy from the Chakra as you breathe out.

4. Now, tell your brain the specific color that corresponds to each individual Chakra. Our consciousness moves faster than the speed of light. If we will the energy of love, our body will be filled with that energy in an instant. If you need healing energy, visualize the golden light of healing... and your aura will immediately shift to the color gold. Create a button inside your brain that you can press to elicit an immediate energy response throughout your body.

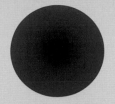

1 First Chakra: **Light of Passion**

Bright, solid red symbolizes strength of life force energy. Red is also the color of the earth, which is the source of all other earth energies. Focus on the first Chakra and commune with her energy for the strength to forgive and the will to be courageous. You will acknowledge and love yourself, with overwhelming passion for life. This passion will make you shine brightly in this reality.

Passion... Courage... Strength... Decisiveness... Forgiveness...
Call forth these fundamental energies to the Hwe-um.
Feel the energies seep into your being.
"I live life with a passion."
"I have courage and strength."
"I am decisive and forgiving."
Breathe in... and out... concentrate on the Hwe-um.
Breathe in, and the red energy comes into you through the Hwe-um.
Breathe out, and the red energy goes out through the Hwe-um.
With the breath, you feel the crimson energy envelop your body.
"A red rose rises through me,
A wave of red energy
Cresting within my soul."

2 Second Chakra: Light of Creation

Colors from light pink to red symbolize joy and happiness of creation. Ordinarily we don't make the connection between sexual energy and creativity. However, the energies of the second Chakra, when nurtured and developed harmoniously, fuel creativity. One who has an active second Chakra is vigorous, sensitive and has a strong sense of aesthetics. On the other hand, diminished second Chakra activity will lead to the sense that life is mundane, boring, and meaningless. Creativity is not the unique gift of artists. It is the God-given right of all. All human beings have a divine purpose for being on Earth. It is up to you to find yours. When you meet with the Creator within, you will find your purpose and be free. When you seek to draw from the reservoir of creativity in yourself, focus on the second Chakra.

Creativity... Joy... Happiness... Vigor...
Call forth the scarlet energy to your lower Dahn-jon.
"I am overflowing with the inner power of creation."
"My heart flows with currents of vigor."
"I am the creator within."
Fill the sky above with the indescribable beauty of the rising sun,
As it comes over the horizon, bearing the gift of light,
Ever changing and exquisite...
Breathe in... and breathe out... concentrate on your Dahn-jon.
Feel scarlet energy in the air around you,
As it becomes part of your energy body.
"I am overflowing with creativity."
"I realize that I am truly the Creator."
"Energy of joy and happiness flow from me."

3 Third Chakra: Light of Life

The orange of the third Chakra calls forth desire and passion for work. The third Chakra has the strength to control impulse and habit, giving you an opportunity to change them. If you want to stop smoking or are on a weight loss program, then concentrate on the third Chakra. Lack of third Chakra activity will lower the level and duration of your ability to concentrate, leaving you vulnerable to diversions. You may also feel frustrated with the lack of progress in the tasks that you do.

Passion for Life... Will... Action... Concentration...
Call the orange energy to your navel.
As you breathe in... and out...
Feel the clear exuberance of orange melting away pain,
Suffering, and indifference.
Feel the energy of courage, hope, and comfort flowing through you.
"I love my work and my life."
"I am healthy and vital, and filled with energy."
"I live in this moment... in the very now."
"Filled with the heat of energy,
I feel the dazzling light of life shining through me."

4 Fourth Chakra: Light of Love

Golden yellow energy has the power to restore balance to the heart and mind. It is the color of forgiveness, understanding, love, and compassion. Overflowing with sympathy, affection, kindness, and hatred, the fourth Chakra can very easily become tired and worn, for this Chakra has overwhelming power to absorb everything that surrounds it. The fourth Chakra's golden light restores strength and peace very quickly. With use of this Chakra, it becomes easier to be convincing, as it imparts power to "move" other people's minds. The fourth Chakra creates a sense of "we" rather than "I" when dealing with others. If you wish to restore a relationship, focus on the fourth Chakra and envelop your heart with its golden light. When your heart overflows with bright, warm light, imagine yourself reconnecting with the other person.

Understanding... Love... Compassion... Kindness...
Visualize a field of yellow flowers
Swaying as one in the breeze.
Powerful golden energy pierces your chest,
And fills your heart, lungs, and blood with a golden aura.
"I am becoming stronger and stronger."
"I am filled with the power to melt away sadness, loneliness, and
Hatred, in the powerful gentle strength of the golden light."
"My heart radiates golden energy
To the whole world...."

5   Fifth Chakra: Light of Peace

Blue-green color represents inspiration, devotion, peace, and silence. Blue-green is also the color of healing, and the restoration of harmony and balance. Blue-green color has the ability to restore the balance of mind and body. It also helps rid the body of toxins and addictions. When you visualize the blue-green sea or sky, or the color of an emerald, you will feel a calm healing sensation through-out your body. Blue-green also has an ameliorating effect on headaches, anxiety, nervousness, insomnia, and palpitations.

Peace... Harmony... Balance... Healing... Calmness...
Imagine a sky without end,
So blue and so high.
Imagine a sea without depth,
So green and so deep.
"Blue-green energy flows through my neck,
Sounding the voice of my soul,
Soft, deep, and powerful."
"It fills me with peace,
That remains still and eternal,
Harmonious and balanced."
"In harmony, all will complete the healing journey."
"I am connected with the very center of the universe."

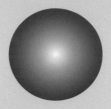

6 Sixth Chakra: **Light of Wisdom**

The sixth Chakra is related to insight and intuition. Insight is not a product of intellect, but rather is the wisdom gained from an understanding of the fundamental truths about life. By silencing your thoughts and preparing your mind, you will be able to meet with the light of the sixth Chakra that connects to the reservoir of wisdom within. The navy blue color of the sixth Chakra will help you expand your awareness and throw off the yoke of fear and repressed emotions. It has a positive effect on diseases of the eyes and ears. It also has an anesthetizing effect. Deep, navy blue will help you expand your awareness, develop intuition and insight, and offer the gift of inspiration.

Insight... Intuition... Wisdom... Inspiration...
The deep, fathomless ocean of wisdom lies within your In-dang.
Feel your body disappear into the silent peace of the deep sea.
Let your body float into the cosmic ocean,
Tethered to your soul with a line of dark blue energy.
"I inhale the light of wisdom, truth, and divinity."
"I exhale with inspiration, intuition, and insight."
"I can hear the voice of wisdom within."
"I can feel the breath of Truth."
"I can breathe the light of divinity."

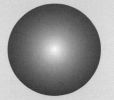

7 Seventh Chakra: Light of Completion

The seventh Chakra is the place where all that has been previously separated comes together in Oneness. You and me... life and death... mind and body... man and woman... all of these melt into the large pot of life. With unshakeable trust in our own divinity, we experience our eternal nature. When we realize our own divinity, we also recognize that fear, loneliness, and other emotions are illusions. Once we rip open the curtain of illusions, we will receive dazzling inspiration and insight. The light of the seventh Chakra will lead us to that place of completion, the place of cosmic divinity. The lavender light of the seventh Chakra symbolizes respect for life and the sacredness of life.

Completion... Oneness... Freedom of Soul...
Whenever you wish... You can will this lavender light to enter you
Through the crown of your head...
"All-knowing and filled with original completeness,
I am perfect and complete and embraced by the light."
"I am neither man nor woman."
"I am neither good nor evil."
"I am eternal and free."
"As I breathe in... and out...
All the separateness I feel becomes one."

2. Exercises to Awaken the Chakras

Chakra exercises are designed to facilitate the flow of energy throughout the body by stimulating the associated meridians. The following exercises help to locate and consciously feel the individual Chakras. These exercises will help you develop a sense of Healing Chakra if practiced prior to training.

First Chakra When seeking strength, courage, and decisiveness

【Contraction/Relaxation Exercise with the Sphincter Muscle】

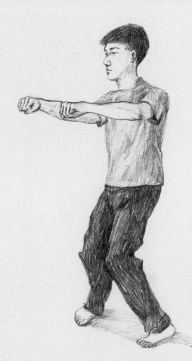

❶ Stand with your legs shoulder width apart and bring your knees together, leaving a space the size of a fist between your right and left knees. Raise your arms straight out in front of you. Straighten your back and hips.

❷ As you breathe in, expand your abdomen and bring your thighs toward the middle while tightening your sphincter muscle. At the same time, make your hands into fists. Then pause.

❸ Breathe out, while you relax your sphincter muscle and suck your abdomen in. Repeat this exercise for ten minutes in the morning and evening.

【Exercise to Stimulate the Hwe-um】

❶ Sit in a butterfly position and grab your ankles with both hands.

❷ Raise your hips up and down so that your Hwe-um area is stimulated. Repeat ten times.

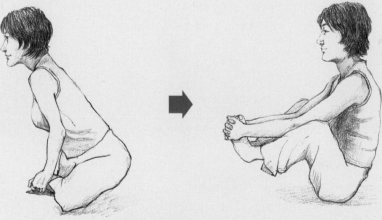

When seeking creativity

【Exercise to Stimulate the Dahn-jon and Kidneys】

❶ Lie on your stomach with your arms to the sides.
Point your toes. Raise your right leg straight up
without bending your knees as you breathe in.
Then, lower your leg slowly as you breathe out.
Repeat this with your left leg.

❷ Once you are accustomed to the exercise, repeat
the above motion with both legs at the same time.

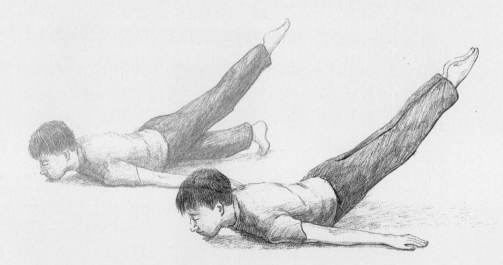

【Exercise to Strengthen the Dahn-jon】

❶ Lie flat on your back. Place your hands behind your head and interlock your fingers. Raise your knees and bring your heels toward your hips.

❷ Breathe in and raise your back up, bringing your knees together and tightening your hips.

❸ Breathe out and lower your back. Repeat this motion three times.

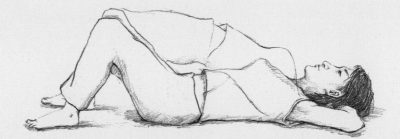

When seeking inner will and desire

【Exercise to Strengthen the Stomach】

❶ Sit in half lotus position with your right leg on top
and place your right hand on top of your right
foot. Breathe in and raise your left arm skyward
while looking at the back of your left hand.

❷ Lower your hand as your breathe out. Repeat with
the other hand. Continue for ten minutes.

【Exercise to Strengthen the Internal Organs】

❶ Lie on your stomach and raise your upper body by pushing up with your arms. With your toes pushing against the floor, breathe in and pull your upper body up and back as far as it will go. As you breathe out, relax.

❷ This time, as you breathe in, tighten your whole body, including your toes until they are off the ground. Breathe out and relax. Raising your legs just a little bit stimulates your digestive organs a great deal.

❸ When doing this exercise, concentrate on the parts of your body that are being worked, including your abdominal area and legs. This exercise stretches the front abdominal and quadriceps areas, stimulating the meridians related to digestion. Repeat 6-8 times daily.

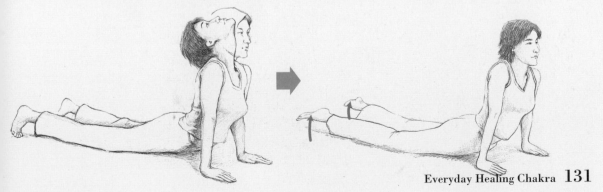

When seeking relief from anxiety and nervousness

【Exercise to Expand the Chest】

❶ Bring your hands together in front of your chest and make them into fists.

❷ As you breathe in, pull your arms back and expand your chest as much as possible. Keep your head back slightly and your back straight, with a slight tightening of your shoulders and chest. Pause for 10 seconds.

❸ Breathe out and bring your hands together in front of your chest again as you bend forward a little. Repeat this motion 10 times. This exercise will bring a refreshing feeling to your chest and shoulders, while relieving stress. You will also feel your mind recover comfort and peace.

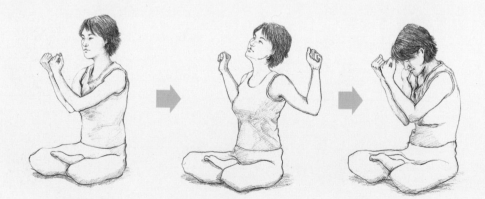

【Exercise to Strengthen the Lungs】

❶ Stand with your legs wide open, knees slightly bent, and lift your arms toward the sky, palms facing upward.

❷ Straighten your back, spine, and chest. Tighten your chest and shoulder muscles as you breathe naturally. In the beginning, hold this position for 5 minutes, then expand the time to 10-20 minutes. This exercise helps you to increase the flow of energy to your lungs by stimulating the relevant points on the spine.

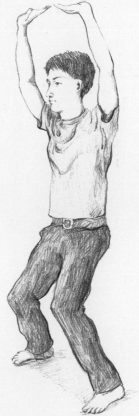

When seeking emotional control and inner peace

【Exercise to Strengthen the Thyroid】

❶ With your hands on your thighs, step one leg forward and the other leg back. Your front leg should be bent at the knee, the back leg straight.

❷ Breathe in as you tilt your head backward, stretching your neck.

❸ Breathe out and bring your head back to its original position. Repeat this motion three times. Also try this with your legs switched.

【Bending the Upper Body】

1 Kneel with your hips resting on your heels. Place both hands on your back, approximately where your kidneys are located.

2 Breathe in and bend your upper body backward as much as possible.

3 Breathe out and bend your back and head forward. Pull your chin down so that it touches your chest.

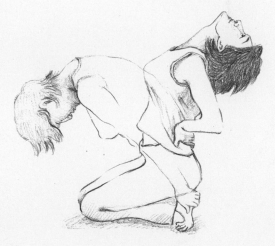

When seeking intuition, inspiration, and insight

【Tae Yang Shin Gong Position to Awaken the 'Third Eye'】

❶ Stand with your legs spread wide and bend your knees about 15 degrees.

❷ Make a triangle by touching your thumbs and index fingers and place it over your In-dang point in your forehead. Breathing naturally, visualize the energy of the sun entering through the triangle into your In-dang. Direct your gaze abut 15 degrees skyward. Continue for five minutes.

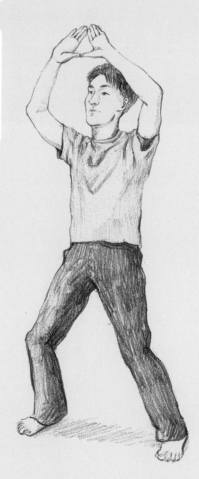

【Exercise to Stimulate the Temples】

❶ Sit comfortably with your eyes closed. Bring one open hand up close to your temple. Will the flow of energy to travel from your hand to your temple.

❷ The other hand should be at the Myung Moon point in your lower back, with the middle finger and the thumb touching in a loop. Imagine breathing through the Myung Moon. The thumb is connected to lower Dahn-jon energy, while the middle finger is connected to upper Dahn-jon energy. The loop facilitates intermingling of the energies.

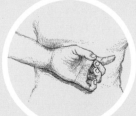
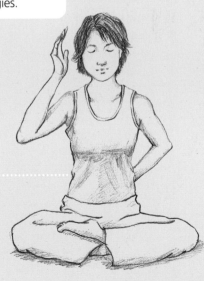

Oneness with the fundamental energy of the cosmos

【Pyramid Position】

❶ Bring the five fingers of each hand together to form a pyramid like shape. The pyramid represents a very stable form of energy. Place the pyramid shape on top of your Baek-hwe. Raise your chin about 15 degrees skyward.

❷ Kneel with your knees touching, back straight, and your feet overlapping. If overlapping the entire foot is difficult, just overlap the big toes.

❸ Breathe naturally for 3-5 minutes and feel the flow of energy throughout your body.

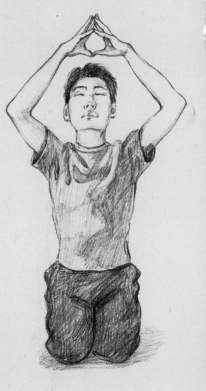

【Lotus Position】

❶ Sit comfortably in half lotus position and focus on your mind. Raise both hands and gradually bring them to your forehead, leaving a little space in between. Focus on the feeling that comes alive between your hands.

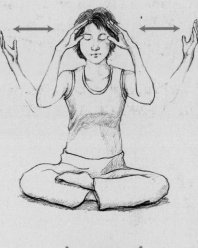

❷ Slowly expand and contract the space between your hands. Imagine your hands as a lotus flower, petals blossoming when you pull your hands apart, and contracting into a bud when you bring your hands together.

❸ Breathe slowly, as you sweep down with your hands from your head to your lower abdomen. Focus on your lower abdomen and continue with the meditation.

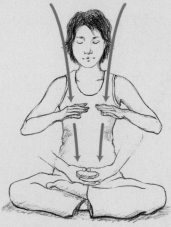

Guide to the Healing Chakra
Self-Training CD and Booklet

**❶ How to use the Healing Chakra
Self -Training CD**

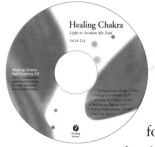

The Healing Chakra CD is for individual use, with one training session per track. You may choose to train by completing one track per session, or you may prefer to complete the whole CD training in one session. This will take about forty minutes. It is a good idea to read and become familiar with the contents of the main Healing Chakra book beforehand.

Tracks 1 and 5 consist of Healing Chakra messages by Ilchi Lee, the creator of Healing Chakra training, recorded in his own voice.

Track 2, "Feeling Your Chakras," is designed to help you identify the exact locations of the Chakras. Following this, you will use the power of music, from the flute, drum, harp and other instruments, to expand the sensation.

Track 3, "Activating the Chakras," is an exercise to help you activate and awaken the seven Chakras through Self-vibration meditation.

Track 4, "Purifying the Chakras," is an exercise to help you cleanse and strengthen your Chakra system. Through the flute music, performed by Ilchi Lee, you can purify and strengthen the

Chakras one by one.

In an impromptu performance, author and musician Ilchi Lee creates music while riding on a wave of the fundamental rhythm of the universe. The result is a powerful healing and soothing effect on the listener.

(List of instruments used: Yullyo Flute, Indian Flute, Native American Drums, Auto Harp, Vibratone, Rain Stick.)

❷ How to use the Healing Chakra Self-Training Booklet

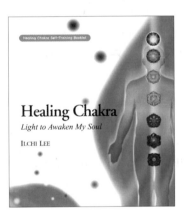

Healing Chakra Brain Respiration is a training method to awaken the infinite possibilities of the brain by activating the Chakras using colors. We will use the unique vibration of each color to stimulate individual Chakras. This in turn stimulates the brain. You can use this training booklet to assist in regular Healing Chakra training or to focus on strengthening a specific Chakra and its associated characteristics. You will enjoy increased energy and alleviate tension and stress by focusing on each Chakra, one at a time.

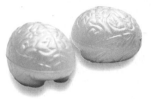

With regular application of vibration, the Power Brain Energizer will stimulate individual Chakras and associated areas of the brain. The Power Brain Energizer is portable, fitting snugly in your hands, to be used at any time and in any place. Its golden brain appearance can be helpful for your visualization. The Power Brain Energizer's soft vibration will soothe your brain waves and activate your Chakras, thereby enhancing your sensitivity to energy.

To find out more information about the Power Brain Energizer, contact *1-877-DAHNHAK* or visit *www.BrainRespiration.com.*